YOGALOSOPHY

for INNER STRENGTH

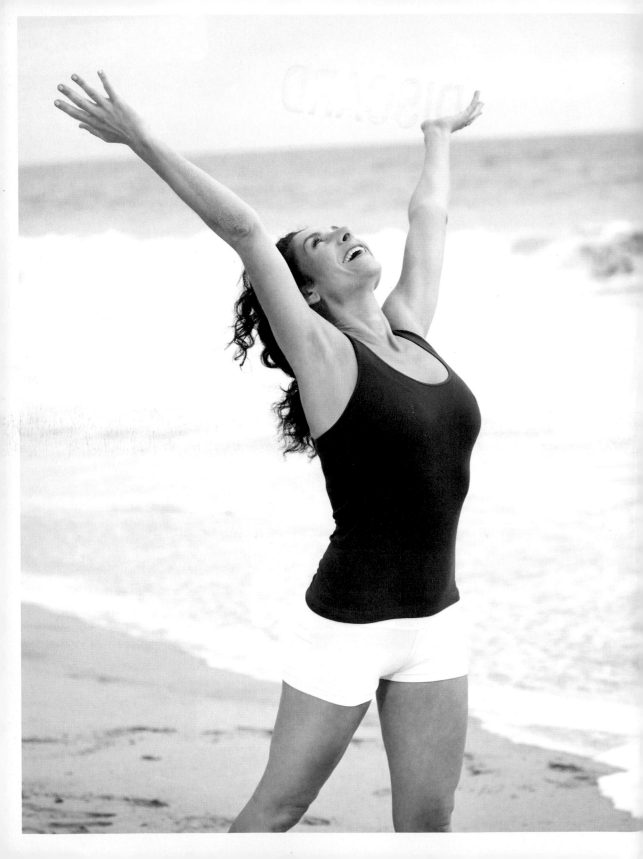

MANDY INGBER

YOGALOSOPHY

for INNER STRENGTH

12 WEEKS *to* HEAL YOUR HEART
and EMBRACE JOY

SEAL PRESS

ISBN 978-1-58005-593-2

Library of Congress Cataloging-in-Publication Data

Names: Ingber, Mandy.
Title: Yogalosophy for inner strength : 12 weeks to heal the heart and
    embrace joy / Mandy Ingber.
Description: Berkeley, California : Seal Press, 2016. | Includes index.
Identifiers: LCCN 2015040213 | ISBN 9781580055932
Subjects: LCSH: Yoga--Philosophy. | Physical fitness. | Mind and body.
Classification: LCC RA781.67 .I55 2016 | DDC 613.7/046--dc23
LC record available at http://lccn.loc.gov/2015040213

Published by
Seal Press
A Member of the Perseus Books Group
1700 Fourth Street
Berkeley, California
Sealpress.com

Cover design by Emily Weigel, Faceout Studio
Cover and interior photography © Javiera Estrada Photography
Heart Chakra image page 166 © Condryx / Getty Images
Photo page 292 © Heather Goldsworthy / Alamy Stock Photo
Chakra icons on page 14 © BerSonnE / istockphoto.com
Interior design by meganjonesdesign.com
Interior production by Domini Dragoone and Tabitha Lahr

Printed in China by RR Donnelley
Distributed by Publishers Group West

This book is dedicated to the mystery.

CONTENTS

PART ONE   *Moving Through Heartbreak*

PART TWO   *The Weekly Companion to Emotional Wellness*

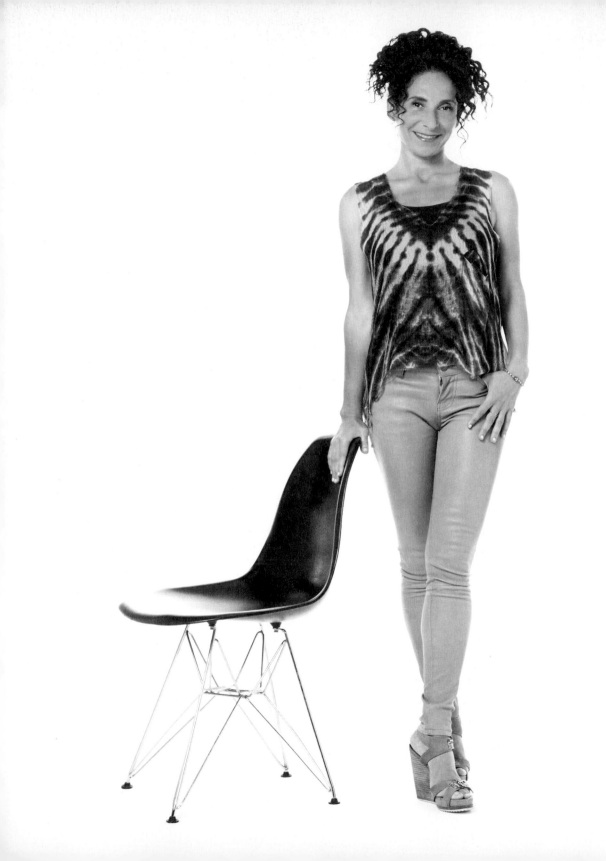

INTRODUCTION

After any type of heartbreak, be it romantic, familial, or otherwise, y
likely to feel a wide range of emotions. You might feel
but directionless, a sense of freedom, deeply
or take a physical step forward. Sometimes multiple
anticipation, anger, despair—coexist at the same time. T
responses as there are individuals, and these undulating
can feel all-consuming, overwhelming, paralyzing, depre
out on your own.

I wrote this book to be your life raft. Within its pages, I will take you on an in-timate, twelve-week journey that will use physical and mental exercises to integrate your diverse emotions and help you develop a new, healing relationship with your heart. That's not to say there's a time frame for grief, like twelve weeks and you're good to go. The path to emotional wellness is an ongoing process—you can't rush it. I know this firsthand because it took me almost five years to fully recover from my first broken heart, and I'm still recovering from my last relationship—and that's after a solid year apart. But I found that a schedule and framework for the journey, which is what this book provides, help focus emotional energy in a particular direction, and that twelve weeks is enough time to learn how to tap into a self-love that will carry you through. No matter how you're feeling right now, you can take action, and those actions will create new thinking. I promise.

If you're feeling crushed, this might seem like an impossible idea, but it is not only possible to achieve—through directing your emotions and using them to fuel actions—it is entirely doable *and* completely transforming.

might be nice to know you're not alone in your plight. Heartbreak is a xperience, and no one has the luxury of avoiding it, including my clients, vell known for their successful careers and their runway-worthy bodies. elebrity and "having it all" doesn't exempt you from pain. There is no fast allows you to skip being human. My client and friend Jennifer Aniston had he most famous and scrutinized breakups on the planet. She credits our work lping her get through it and discovering that she could *act her way into correct* . Jennifer is living evidence that moving your body with heart produces the onal result you're looking for. Using her emotional energy positively has trans-d her. She has reached an entirely new level of personal power and comfort in her own skin. I hold very dearly the very first time we practiced yoga together. It was a devastating time, when she was exposed to more pain than most of us with a freshly wounded heart can handle, and I suggested that we simply move the energy with some yoga. I let her know that if she needed more energy she could tap into what she was feeling, and if that didn't do it, she could tap into me. That is what I suggest to you, too, through this book.

Jennifer isn't the only one who found her way to me at a devastating time. Many of my students first came to my class or began working with me during a difficult life phase. While many can become paralyzed by mourning and find it difficult to take a physical step forward, others, sometimes unknowingly, seek to find a way to release some of the pent-up grief by taking a yoga class. Perhaps intuitively they know that one of the best things you can do to help yourself heal is to find action-oriented ways to love yourself through physical movement. As an instructor, I've found that once people get into the routine of showing up for themselves, the endorphins kick in and they want to come back for more of that good feeling. Consequently, they end up getting in the best shape of their lives—while healing the emotional body, too.

The practices in this book are distinct from my first book, *Yogalosophy: 28 Days to the Ultimate Mind-Body Makeover*, in an important way. There I talk about emotion being a motivating force: take your emotion and change your body with it. Here, we flip that dynamic to discover how you can shift your emotions by getting physical—and conversely, change your thinking by fully expressing your feelings through action too. and movement. There's a saying—"Move a muscle, change a thought"—that perfectly reflects this dynamic.

So here we are. At your new beginning. Follow this book and I guarantee you'll change your thoughts, your habits, and your body. But before we dive in, I want to share a bit about myself and my experience. This is something I'll do throughout these pages because opening up and relating my personal experiences has always been key to my teaching—whether in my classes, with my private clients, through my DVD, or in my first book, *Yogalosophy: 28 Days to the Ultimate Mind-Body Makeover*. In the deeply personal arena of heartbreak, I will allow you inside my own journey as it speaks to each of the movements in the twelve-week process. Sharing is a way of teaching and also of learning. Instead of the feeling of isolation that often accompanies sadness, we can open ourselves up and widen our circle. In this sharing I also want to explain a bit about how this book works, so once you get into the twelve weeks you'll know what to expect.

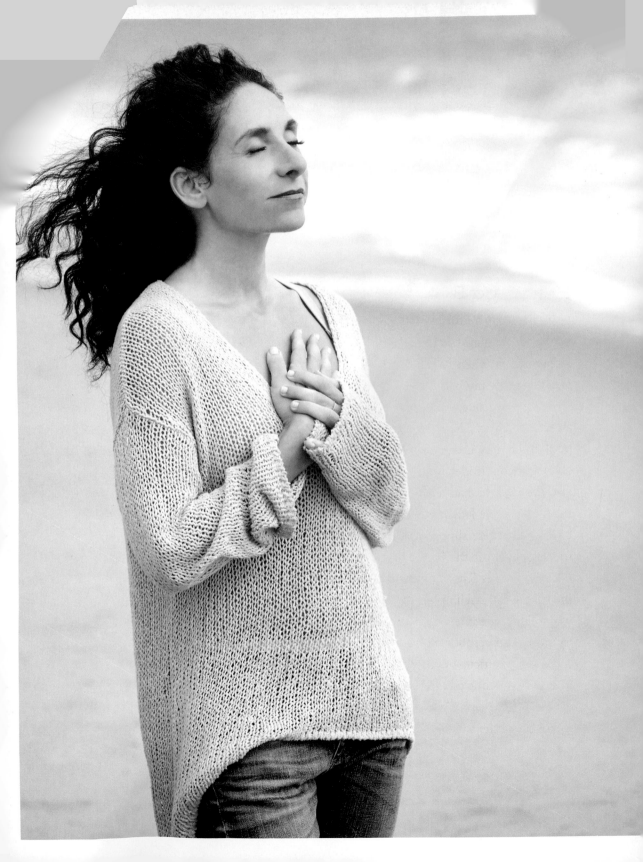

OVERVIEW

How Yoga Broke My Heart Wide Open

Let me tell you a little secret. I kind of hate yoga. You might think I'm kidding, but I'm not. Well, *sort* of not. Yoga caused my first heartbreak. Yoga represented the breakdown of my family when I was a child. It's ironic that *yoga* means "union"—considering it was what tore my parents apart.

On the outside, we appeared to be the perfect family. My parents were attractive and charismatic. They had two kids, myself and my brother, and a nice home with a pool in the ritzy Los Angeles neighborhood of Bel Air. My mom was a dedicated parent, Girl Scout leader, and everyone's listening ear. My father was an attorney. He was also a seeker; he had a knack for discovering things about thirty years ahead of their time. It was the late seventies when Dad found yoga and a macrobiotic diet. After a bout with severe slipped discs, which had him flat on his back for over a month, a friend of his from the gym, actor Dirk Benedict (to date myself, he was from the 1970s television series *Battlestar Galactica*), introduced him to a macrobiotic diet and told him that yoga and cycling would heal his back. It was the beginning of a journey that would last a lifetime, and would make my mother a slave to the kitchen, whipping up four-course macrobiotic meals—no easy task.

We were strict—not merely avoiding certain foods, but also using food as medicine. In the macrobiotic tradition, the head of the household—my mother—was in charge of getting a bead on how to best balance each family member's condition, reading characteristics of the tongue, the face (using physiognomy), and the eyes (using iridology). My mother was responsible for this diagnosing and then preparing the appropriate foods in the appropriate ways, based on the principles of Yin and Yang. This was much more than "dairy free," "gluten free," or "vegetarian"; this was a complete lifestyle overhaul. My mother still tells the story about when she took my brother, David, and myself to the market and showed us the section we would be able to select food from, and how we burst into tears. Thank goodness for the moments of levity when Mom used her wooden spoons to break into an outstanding Mick Jagger impression while preparing brown rice in a pressure cooker, or when we would read stories to her in different accents while she was making tempura!

My parents' arguing had always been an issue, and now some of it surrounded yoga, health, and wellness. It's no wonder that I became averse to sitting down to meals with the family. But I wasn't the only one. Each of us, with our own separate way of eating, was on our own. Soon, my father was eating in a kneeling position at the head of the dining room table all by himself. My brother, vegged out in front of the television with his nonvegetarian Stouffer's frozen dinners. And my mom ate out of the pots she was cooking from, scraping the pan, delighting in the extra flavor of the burnt morsels at the bottom.

I preferred to stay out of it entirely. Due to the family dynamics and my own need for control, I survived on very little. I distinctly remember using the cap of a white grape juice bottle to enjoy a thimbleful of the sweet elixir after a day or two of starvation. In an effort to gain my father's attention, I began to practice from B. K. S. Iyengar's *Light on Yoga*, just as he did. My flexibility, although inherited from him, impressed my father. My efforts to practice and expand my knowledge of yoga came from a competitive place, one that stemmed from a deep admiration of and longing for my father's approval.

As my folks continued to contract and expand around these lifestyle issues, I contracted into eating disorders and expanded into my imagination to become an actress. Perhaps, I thought, if I eliminated food entirely from the plate, there would be no conflict in my world. Everybody would leave me alone. My brother found his individuality in the art and drug scene, and my family seemed to be unyoking. Meanwhile, my father's expansion into more esoteric yogic practices led him into the arms of another woman, Alex. She was not only the mother of one of my friends at school but she was also my dad's "yoga buddy." Alex and dad were two peas in a pod, practicing yoga and exploring their spirituality together. And when my father would feel a spasm at "the left tip of my right kidney," she concurred—he was so deeply enamored of her he even thought she was able to see into his internal organs. They were like two aliens dropped onto planet Earth and into the "body experiment." My mother was left crying over the loss of the only thing she had ever been raised to do: get married and have children. Be a family. This was no longer an option. She sobbed for months on end. Looking back, I am so grateful that she allowed me to see and hear her tears. But at the time, I was a sixteen-year-old girl. I was on the brink of embarking on life as a young woman, and I had spent most of my years witnessing the deterioration of a relationship. I wanted to get some space from my parents' woes.

And so I developed a love-hate relationship with yoga. Is it any wonder? There was no yoga community like there is today to turn to, but what was there was related to my father and his newfound partner, so I often felt isolated. As a result, I practiced the yoga positions halfheartedly, never really feeling that they were my own, but rather a shadow of my family that I was trying to hang on to.

> *"Yoga has helped me accept that the cracks in my heart are the openings where the light shines through."*

The irony doesn't escape me that my family broke up over yoga while so many people turn to it to attain wholeness. But I have learned that, like homeopathy, the cure is often in the poison.

As I grew older and experienced my first romantic heartbreak, I found that the antidote to my hurt was contained within yoga. After my first big break-up, I signed up for a yoga teacher's training and immersed myself in the studies, physical action, and ritual of the yoga practice. But yoga classes felt like a haunted house to me. Each woman that I saw in the class had the potential to be "the other woman." In fact, one of the teachers who trained me actually *had* slept with my ex-boyfriend. My nightmare *did* come true, over and over again. Now I don't see this so much as coincidence as it was my path. Life tends to open the old wounds as it presents us with circumstances that cut straight to the bone—which ache like original betrayal—in order for us to view them and heal from them from a new, empowered position. My journey with yoga has been a way of reclaiming myself by moving toward the pain of heartbreak and finding the wisdom in the broken-openness. Yoga has helped me accept that the cracks in my heart are openings where the light shines through. They leave me vulnerable and allow me to be truly seen, whether I like it or not. The process of going in deeper and leaning in toward the pain is a constant practice in yoga that requires patience. It cannot be forced; if it is, it can set you back. Yet if discomfort is avoided completely, growth and change will remain untapped. But meeting myself at the edge of my pain—without force, without avoidance—is a place of sweetness. It reminds me that I am human. It reminds me that this, too, shall pass, and that I am equally capable of love and loss. And that when I lean into the pain, and can be with it, there is bliss just on the other side of that threshold.

How to Use This Book

You don't need to know anything about yoga to make it through the next twelve weeks. All you need to do is read one chapter per week in Part 2: The Weekly Companion to Emotional Wellness. Then follow the included physical and mental/emotional exercises, which are meant both to align your heart and body and to tap into two of the main concepts in yogic tradition—the eight limbs of yoga and the chakra system. (I will further explain these in Part 1: Moving Through Heartbreak.)

At the core of this book's weekly plans are five Yogalosophy-inspired routines. If they are unfamiliar to you, don't worry. I've included photos and descriptions of the poses in the upcoming Moving Through Heartbreak section. You'll do one of these routines each day for five days, plus cardio for an additional day.

In addition to these routines, in Part 1 you'll also find a nutritional support section called Eat Your Heart Out! because there is a close connection between what you eat and how you feel. I'm not putting you on a diet. It's enough that you are experiencing a fundamental loss, so the point is not to take away anything else. There are, however, foods that support your heart and make you feel better. Eating cleanly will allow you to attain more emotional balance. For example, sugar can be a comfort, but it is not your friend when you're looking for stability.

You'll also find basic food guidelines for emotional wellness, which will help you to eat whole foods, hydrate, avoid refined sugars and processed foods, fuel up with protein for breakfast, and experience pleasure through daily nutritious, delicious treats.

Along with a weekly routine of yoga and healthful eating, each week focuses on healing various elements of your heart through the following practices, which you'll find at the end of each chapter.

MANTRA: This is your weekly affirmation to help put your mind and emotional body in the right space.

TRACK OF THE WEEK: Music helps you access your emotions and touches the intangible spirit that connects us all. This track is meant to evoke the theme of the week on an emotional and spiritual level.

HEART-OPENING POSE: Each pose includes accompaniment, instruction, and reflective text that relates to the theme of the week.

LOVE MOVEMENT: This is your weekly cardiovascular activity to strengthen your heart and keep your energy in motion.

HEART-HEALING MEDITATION: This is your weekly meditation or breathing exercise to bring clarity and harness the mind.

LOVE NOTES: This is a weekly topical journal or writing exercise for expressing emotions on the page.

RITUAL: Powerful actions help to express and release emotion through ritual. This can be a real catalyst for change.

STRENGTH FOR THE SOUL: This section offers a mixed bag of food lists, self-care suggestions, playlists, and activities that connect you with others.

HEART FACT: For your information, a fun fact about the heart.

HEART-HEALTHY TREAT: Eat your heart out with a special food item, recipe, or "treat" related to the theme of the week.

Along the way, you'll also find stories and recipes or other remedies from my circle of women, who are experts in their fields and have greatly impacted me with their wisdom and experience. My contributors are strong women. Nutritionists, chefs, daughters, mothers, friends, teachers, jewelry makers, artists, yoginis, actors—women just like you and me who have come to know that each loss has brought with it a blessing. When we share our stories, we heal together, and create a network of love that unifies us all. Join us here. Share with us in the bittersweet beauty that connects and softens us all: vulnerability. I would like to invite you into this sacred circle. Heartbreak is a turning point where we get to choose what we do with the broken-openness—and that choice is how we take part in writing our story. We are each different and pull wisdom from one another.

As you move forward in this process, remember that you can pick and choose what works for you. Though these exercises are tools for you to use as needed, the main idea is to rekindle a love relationship with yourself. You will discover so many new strengths that emerge from self-acceptance, self-love, and simply learning to be present with yourself as you are. I will never forget my father's words of wisdom when my heart was aching with grief. He reminded me that the gifts I would garner from this heartache would far outweigh the gifts of the relationship I had lost. Even through my pain, I heeded his words because I sensed from within that this was true.

PART ONE

Moving Through Heartbreak

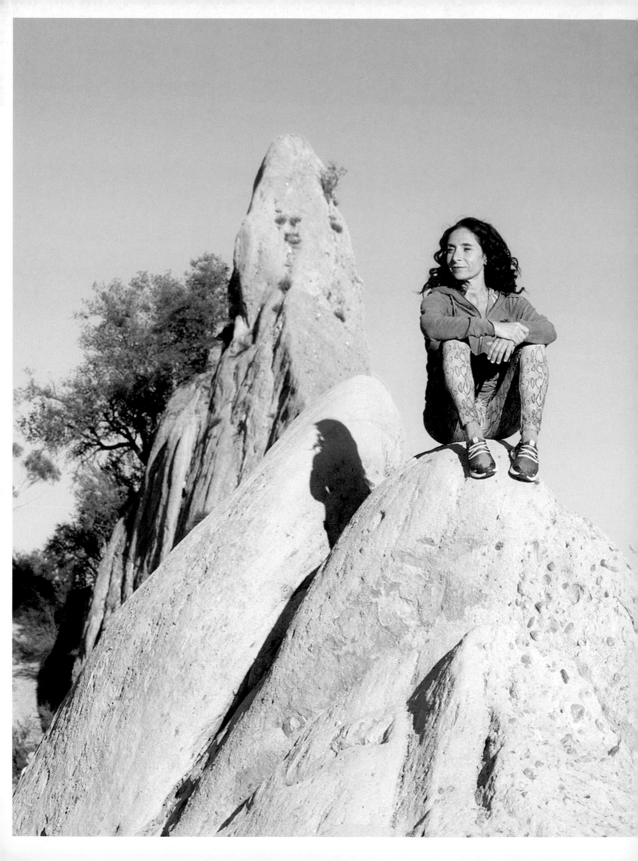

BASICS OF YOGIC TRADITION

The Eight Limbs of Yoga

The Eight Limbs of Yoga, also known as the Eightfold Path, is part of the teachings derived from the Yoga Sutras, as dictated by Patanjali. It is a nonreligious text about how to live in union with the Divine. The word *sutra* translated from Sanskrit means "thread." They are seen as the thread between the knowledge of and the experience of yoga.

Since yoga has been adopted by the West and integrated into our Western lifestyle, it is no surprise that we have focused on the physical aspect of the practice more than any other. The physical practice, *asana,* is just one of the eight limbs! When you see practitioners engaged in a class in a variety of postures, the physical practice is what you are seeing, and that is just a fraction of what the yoga practice addresses. Physicality is a wonderful way to confront issues of the mind and to unwind areas of tension that impede us from more contemplative practices, but there is so much more to it.

The eightfold path is as follows:

1. Ethical standards relating to others (Nonviolence, Truthfulness, Nonstealing, Abstinence, Nonhoarding)

2. Ethical standards relating to self (Cleanliness; Contentment; Heat, spiritual sternness, to burn; Study of text and self; Surrender)

3. Postures

4. Therapeutic breathing

5. Withdrawal of the senses

6. Concentration

7. Meditation

8. Absorption with the universe

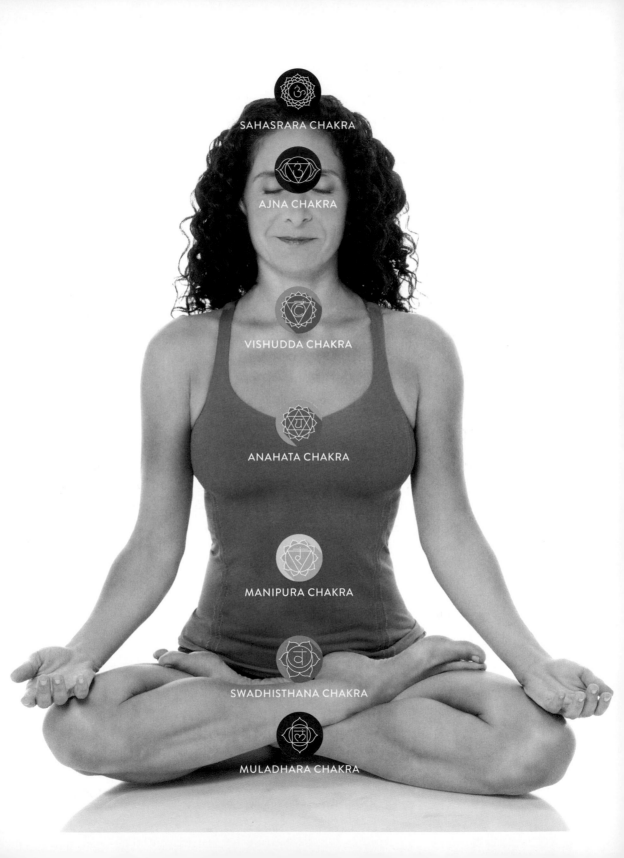

SAHASRARA CHAKRA

AJNA CHAKRA

VISHUDDA CHAKRA

ANAHATA CHAKRA

MANIPURA CHAKRA

SWADHISTHANA CHAKRA

MULADHARA CHAKRA

The Seven Chakras

Yogic tradition believes in energy bodies, that we are not merely physical. When you have a holistic yoga practice, you address multiple layers of that energy field in order to awaken and enliven the energy centers that exist in your subtle body. These wheels of light are called chakras. The word *chakra* means "turning" or "wheel" in Sanskrit, and refers to the vortex-like energy center in and beyond the flesh. They store all our energy and life force, which is also called *prana*. The release of this energy is controlled by the breath. The seven major chakras are located on the chief energy path, called the *sushumna*, that runs up the spine. There are two sides to this column, one governing the masculine principle and the other governing the feminine principle. These are not gender-based—they are simply qualities contained within each of us. Yoga postures and breathing techniques can help to keep the polarity of masculine and feminine, also known as Yang and Yin, in harmonious balance. To follow is a brief reference point for each chakra and what part of the self each affects.

 ## ROOT CHAKRA (*Muladhara*)

Located at the sacral center, the root chakra is connected to our survival and creativity and is concerned with such basics as food, shelter, and staying alive. The first chakra grounds and connects us to the Earth. The root, located at the base of the tailbone, is the basis for creativity and self-expression.

COLOR: Red

MANTRA: "I have"

ELEMENT: Earth

SOUND: *Lam*

PHYSICAL ASPECT: Anus, genitals, feet, legs, sacrum

MENTAL AND EMOTIONAL ASPECT: Family ties and all our relations (to the planet, tribe, etc.). Feelings of the basic needs of survival and belonging. Providing for ourselves, our sense of safety in the world. If we have a strong root chakra, we have the confidence to stand up and take care of ourselves. When it is blocked or out of balance, we may feel needy, have low self-esteem, or have self-destructive tendencies.

SACRAL CHAKRA (*Swadhisthana*)

Located at the pelvic region, the second chakra is experienced through sexuality and how we relate with others. It is creativity and helps us to understand how our emotional/mental states affect us. When empowered, it honors our intuitive nature and allows us to be receptive and intimate.

COLOR: Orange

MANTRA: "I feel"

ELEMENT: Water

SOUND: *Vam*

PHYSICAL ASPECT: Reproductive sexual organs, lower back, hips

MENTAL AND EMOTIONAL ASPECT: Feeling deserving of pleasure, creativity, and abundance. Literally, the themes of sex, money, power, relationships, truth telling, creativity, and procreativity are at play. When it is out of balance, it rises in the form of emotional instability, especially in being hard on ourselves.

SOLAR PLEXUS CHAKRA (*Manipura*)

Located at the solar plexus center, the third chakra is related to the "I am": identity and willpower. It helps us to stand up for ourselves. It gives us the ability to think and reason, feeling the knowing from our gut. It is connected to the umbilical cord and the original cell in the body. When healthy, the third chakra allows us to get clarity of the mind while allowing fun, play, liveliness, and pleasure with a positive, childlike innocence.

COLOR: Yellow

MANTRA: "I do"

ELEMENT: Fire

SOUND: *Ram*

PHYSICAL ASPECT: Abdominal wall, chain of obliques, thoracic spine

MENTAL AND EMOTIONAL ASPECT: Gives a sense of self-esteem and allows us to take action. Key words are: gut feelings, backbone, standing up for one's self, navel center, umbilical cord, digesting life. This gives us a sense of inner power (willpower) and helps us to take risks. When it is blocked, it can read as lacking courage and feeling stuck.

 ## HEART CHAKRA (*Anahata*)

Located at the heart, the fourth chakra has the quality of compassion. It gives us vitality for being alive and allows us to feel for others—to be truly connected and interested. And as it is the pathway from the body to the mind, feeling and unconditional love are the gateway from the lower realms to the higher realms.

COLOR: Green

MANTRA: "I love"

ELEMENT: Air

SOUND: *Yam*

PHYSICAL ASPECT: Heart, shoulders, clavicle, arms, hands

MENTAL AND EMOTIONAL ASPECT: A healthy heart chakra allows feelings of unconditional love, compassion, forgiveness, and acceptance. It is the highway between the animal self and divine self; in other words, the heart keeps the balance and allows us to be in healthy relationships. Due to fear of rejection, a blocked heart chakra is isolated and can become possessive or codependent.

 ## THROAT CHAKRA (*Vishudda*)

Located at the throat, the fifth chakra revolves around speaking your truth, which comes from the higher self. Communication, self-expression, imagination, and

ease in communicating our needs (especially during transitions and life changes) are its territory. Singing or chanting can be a wonderful way to connect with this chakra.

COLOR: Blue

MANTRA: "I speak"

ELEMENT: Ether

SOUND: *Ham*

PHYSICAL ASPECT: Throat, neck, occipital lobes, jaw

MENTAL AND EMOTIONAL ASPECT: Speaking your true inner voice. It includes speaking up for the self, voice, and aligning the human will with the Divine will (as in "Thy will be done"). When aligned, this chakra allows clear communication of the emotions in speaking and listening. When blocked, you may have trouble by being too verbal or not being able to listen to others.

THIRD EYE CHAKRA (*Ajna*)

Located between the brows, the sixth chakra is connected to "knowing or intuition," otherwise known as the "sixth sense." This chakra allows insight and calls to your inner guidance. This is a spiritual energy center and deepens your connection to a higher calling. It knows intuitively in the silence.

COLOR: Indigo

MANTRA: "I see"

ELEMENT: Light

SOUND: *Om*

PHYSICAL ASPECT: Between eyes, ears, center of head

MENTAL AND EMOTIONAL ASPECT: Intuition, night vision, foresight, cellular-level knowledge, silence. It governs all of the other chakras and aids in trusting our inner wisdom to face life on life's terms. When it is blocked, we can be too serious, with an overbearing logic, lack of trust, and cynicism.

CROWN CHAKRA (*Sahasrara*)

Located at the crown (which is open at the top of the head when you enter the world!), the crown chakra is true awareness and helps you to stretch beyond self-imposed limitations. This chakra gives understanding and the ability to expand into new ways of being. It is devotion, prayer, and surrender.

COLOR: Violet

MANTRA: "I understand"

ELEMENT: Cosmos

PHYSICAL ASPECT: Scalp, head, crown, beyond the actual physical body

MENTAL AND EMOTIONAL ASPECT: Spirit itself. It is ether, devotion, prayer, and surrender. The gift of total freedom. When it is out of balance, you can forget that all is well in the spiritual realm and can think that happiness comes from what you "have" instead of what you are—both of which can cause suffering.

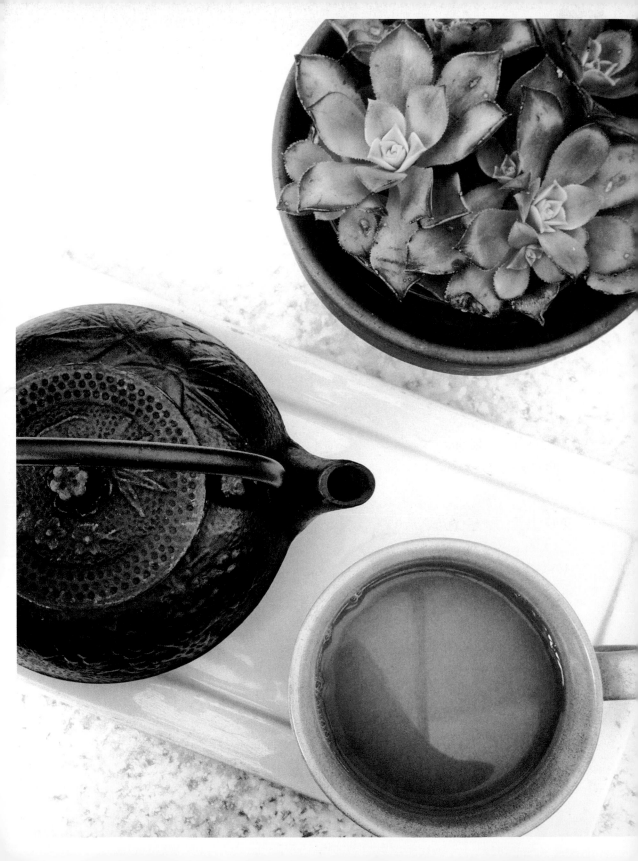

HEART HEALTHY SUPPORT: EAT YOUR HEART OUT!

I know from experience that one of the first things that drops off during a time of loss is one's diet. People often let themselves go, either by not eating (as many of us lose our appetite when grieving) or by drowning their sorrows with emotional eating. Using food as a distraction or to numb emotions is very common. The last thing I want to do is restrict you, but what you put into your body is key to your emotional state. The first thing that I do when experiencing a loss is make sure I'm taking care of my health needs. Since I cannot fully trust my appetite during these times, I take extra care to give myself support for healing. Here are some of my tips.

Mandy's Guidelines for a Healthy Diet

HYDRATE

Increase your intake of water and fluids. By the time you're thirsty, you are already dehydrated. The general rule of thumb is to calculate your body weight, and divide that in half. The number you get is the minimum amount of ounces you should be drinking per day. So if you are 130 pounds, that would be 65 ounces of water. I've actually taken to drinking (in ounces) almost my entire body's weight, meaning I don't divide that number in half. Whatever amount you go with, set aside a 20-ounce glass water bottle and fill it with spring water or filtered water 4 or 5 times a day. Glugging your water down will just go right through you, so instead sip throughout the day. Begin your day with an additional 16 ounces of warm water and lemon. Hydration is the key to your digestion, as it will help your digestive juices and aid proper elimination. It will keep your body metabolizing, and increases your daily calorie burn. Gut health is the foundation to your organs functioning properly and will help you to eliminate any stored toxins. In short, staying hydrated is essential to your health!

EAT AT LEAST FIVE SERVINGS OF FRUITS AND VEGETABLES

Eating at least five servings of fruits and veggies each day is a good guideline for making sure you get enough nutrients and antioxidants in your diet. There are a variety of fruits and vegetables that you can choose from. Select locally grown, organic produce if you can. I love going to the farmer's market because I love knowing my local farmers and where my food is sourced. Avoid genetically modified produce that can be contaminated with pesticides.

EAT DARK LEAFY GREENS FOR DETOXIFICATION

Greens are excellent for your blood, and the darker the better. For those who find it a challenge to work greens into your diet, adding a 16-ounce cold-pressed green juice (all veggie) is the equivalent of two servings of vegetables. I recommend drinking one green juice daily. You may also supplement with Vitamineral Green, or toss a cup of dark leafy greens into your morning smoothie.

NOURISH YOUR BODY EVERY THREE-TO-FOUR HOURS

When you wait too long to fuel your body, your blood sugar levels drop. When this happens you can not only lose energy but also become emotional without realizing why. Set your timer to go off after three hours to make sure that you're taking care of yourself the way you would your own child. You don't want to wait until your child is crying—you want to keep the homeostasis of your body. Each time you recharge yourself, consider it a mini prescription for self-love.

START YOUR DAY WITH A HEARTY BREAKFAST

The first meal of the day sets the tone for your day. Of course, if you are not a morning eater, you must honor that, but do create some sort of ritual around the first meal of the day. If it's got to be quick and light, a smoothie or shake with protein powder is a great way to keep your muscles fed and to give your body foundational support to build upon. I plan my morning meal the night before, sometimes preparing my steel-cut oats by precooking and soaking them overnight for a quick morning prep. I also prepare a to-go container in case I need to rush out of the house. Other quick options: eggs with sliced avocado, or fresh berries with Greek yogurt.

TREAT YOURSELF

Yes, it's important to find the foods that taste like treats to you. There are plenty of them out there these days. Make a list of the foods that are heart healthy *and* that you love to eat. In this book I have included recipes and suggestions for some delicious heart-healthy treats that I enjoy, but feel free to play around with your favorite healthy foods and find your happy place.

ABSTAIN FROM SUGAR AND COFFEE OR FOODS THAT SPIKE YOUR BLOOD SUGAR LEVEL

I have a sweet tooth just like anybody else. Plus, coffee is my on-again/off-again love affair, and it even zoomed me through the grieving period after my father's passing. I will say, though, that each of these stimulants will have you riding above your emotions while offering little nutritional value. This is your choice, and do with them as you will; however, note that restriction or minimal intake of both may help your moods. Just saying.

HEART-HEALTHY FOODS FOR YOUR PANTRY

- almonds
- apples
- artichokes
- asparagus
- avocado
- banana
- blueberries
- black beans
- broccoli
- brown rice
- Brussels sprouts
- cantaloupe
- carrots
- cauliflower
- chia seeds
- dark chocolate
- flaxseed
- grapefruit
- green tea
- kale
- kidney beans
- mackerel
- oatmeal
- olive oil
- oranges
- papaya
- pomegranate
- popcorn
- rainbow trout
- raisins
- red bell peppers
- salmon
- sardines
- spinach
- sweet potato
- tea
- tomatoes
- tuna
- walnuts

ask the expert

I asked registered dietician and nutrition communications professional, **Sarah Romotsky**—who has an extensive background in writing and speaking on health and wellness issues and is a respected leader and spokesperson in the nutrition community—to chime in on nutrition and physical heart health. Knowledge is power, and although the best way to find out what works for you is to listen to your body and discover for yourself, in general, having an expert to guide you toward incorporating these foods into your diet will help give you a starting point.

SARAH'S TOP-FIVE FOODS FOR HEART HEALTH

We all know that keeping your heart healthy is important. This complex organ is literally at the "heart" of all biological functions, circulating blood throughout the body, maintaining blood flow, and regulating cholesterol levels. There are a variety of strategies we can incorporate into our lives to promote heart health, including managing weight and stress, getting regular physical activity and sleep, and maintaining a heart-healthy diet.

You may often hear about "superfoods" that contain heart-healthy benefits, but it's important to remember that superfoods are only "superior" to other foods when there is science behind them. Don't get fooled into the latest trap of the hot new food that is "guaranteed" to improve heart health. As a registered dietitian, I can tell you that there are some foods that have proven associated health benefits and some that are not worth the money. We are always told to "go with your heart" when making decisions, but when it comes to foods with health benefits, I'm here to give you some science to back that up—so you can "go with your head" as well.

Here is my list of the top-five foods to incorporate into your diet to improve your heart health. Backed by research and supported by experts, the following list will help guide you in making these heart-healthy decisions.

HEALTHY FATS IN FISH

After the anti-fat days of the 1980s and '90s, dietary fats have a new lease on life with the compelling research that proves *healthy* fats can positively impact health. These healthy fats include polyunsaturated fats such as omega-3 fatty acids. From salmon to tuna to sardines, fish are a large source of omega-3 fatty acids, including eicosapentaenoic acid and docosahexaenoic acid.

Benefits That Can't Be "Beat"

Research has demonstrated that increased consumption of fish reduces coronary heart disease mortality as well as reduced cardiovascular disease risk factors. Omega-3 fatty acids may also decrease triglyceride levels, slow the growth rate of plaque accumulating in arteries, and slightly lower blood pressure. Omega-3 fatty acids may also lower the risk of developing other diseases such as certain cancers, neurological disorders, and complications from metabolic syndrome and diabetes. Some studies also show an association between omega-3 consumption and improved bone health among older adults, healthy pregnancy outcomes, and good cognitive and visual development among infants.

Eat Your Heart Out

Omega-3 fatty acids can be found in freshwater fatty fish such as herring, salmon, mackerel, and tuna. Fish oils can also be bought in the form of a capsule. You can also get omega-3 fatty acids in nonfish sources such as walnuts, flaxseed oil, soybeans, and canola oil.

To promote cardiovascular health, the American Heart Association recommends at least two servings of fish (or other omega-3 rich foods) per week.

WHOLE GRAINS

Although grains (and carbohydrates in general) may get a bad rap from some, they have rightly earned their place on a heart-healthy plate. Whole grains are unprocessed grains that contain the same relative proportions of endosperm, bran, and germ as found in intact grains. They can be consumed as a single food, such as barley, brown rice, oatmeal, popcorn, or quinoa, used as an ingredient in foods such as whole wheat flour in bread, cereal, or bars. The fiber content of different whole grain foods can vary considerably, depending on the food category and serving size. Refined grains differ from whole grains in that they have been milled to remove the bran and the germ from the grain.

Benefits That Can't Be "Beat"

Eating a diet rich in whole grains may provide many health benefits, including weight management, digestive health, maintaining normal blood glucose levels, and reduced risk of type 2 diabetes. Additionally, studies continue to show that including enough whole grain foods as part of a healthy diet may help with heart disease prevention and management. Researchers have even

observed that diets rich in whole grain foods tend to decrease LDL cholesterol (the "bad" cholesterol), triglycerides, and blood pressure, and increase HDL cholesterol (the "good" cholesterol).

Eat Your Heart Out

There are many different types of whole grains, including whole wheat, whole oats, whole grain
cornmeal, popcorn, brown rice, whole rye, whole grain barley, wild rice, buckwheat, triticale, bulgur
(cracked wheat), millet, quinoa, and sorghum. Other less common whole grains include amaranth,
emmer, farro, grano (lightly pearled wheat), spelt, and wheat berries.

The USDA's Dietary Guidelines for Americans recommend consuming at least half your
grains as whole grains. This means that at least three-ounce equivalents of whole grains per day
are necessary to achieve the dietary recommendation of making half your grains whole.

FRUITS AND VEGETABLES

Of course, it isn't big news to say that fruit and vegetables provide health benefits, but their positive impact on cardiovascular health can't be understated. The key is to have a variety of fruits
and vegetables in your diet so you'll be taking in a range of the important nutrients associated
with heart health. Here are a few examples of different fruits and vegetables and their associated
heart-healthy benefits.

Benefits That Can't Be "Beat"

Tomato: Tomatoes are a rich source of lycopene, a class of antioxidants that has been shown
to promote heart health. Studies have shown a negative correlation between lycopene and
negative heart health outcomes such as arterial stiffness and LDL cholesterol levels.

Berries: Whether it's strawberries, blueberries, or any other type, berries all contain important
antioxidants called polyphenols that promote heart health by increasing good cholesterol and
lowering blood pressure.

Avocado: Full of phytosterols, this versatile food has cholesterol-lowering properties. They are
high in monounsaturated (good) fats and high in fiber. Monounsaturated fats can help reduce
"bad" cholesterol levels in the blood—in addition to lowering your risk for heart disease and stroke.
Avocados also contain potassium, vitamin E, and B vitamins, which are important micronutrients

in the regulation of blood pressure, preventing coronary heart disease and decreasing risk of stroke or heart attack.

Eat Your Heart Out

Dietary Guidelines for Americans recommends filling half your plate with fruits and vegetables. With such a broad recommendation, there are so many ways to fulfill these requirements. The foods listed above are only examples of the myriad of ways fruits and vegetables can have a positive impact on your health.

YOGURT

Packed with so many healthful nutrients, yogurt really is powerhouse food for health. Yogurt is an excellent source of calcium, potassium, and protein and also contains beneficial components called prebiotics and probiotics that maintain a healthy digestive and immune system.

Benefits That Can't Be "Beat"

Although yogurt is most commonly associated with digestive health benefits, studies have shown that it can also play a role in improving cardiovascular health as well. Studies have shown that 100 grams of daily yogurt intake (slightly less than half a cup) protected against heart attack and stroke by preventing plaque buildup in arteries. Research has also found that daily yogurt consumption increased HDL (good) cholesterol levels.

Yogurt is also a complete protein source, meaning it contains all the essential amino acids in the right amount. Dietary protein plays a significant role in overall health and wellness and, more specifically, is linked to improved cardiovascular health, weight management/weight loss, bone health, immune health, and maintenance of lean muscle mass.

Eat Your Heart Out

The Dietary Guidelines for Americans recommend that individuals ages nine and older consume three servings of milk, cheese, or yogurt each day; children of four to eight years old should consume two and a half servings. One serving of yogurt is one eight-ounce cup or container.

NUTS

These crunchy snacks pack a punch since they're loaded with beneficial nutrients and heart-protective fats. They also contain important vitamins and minerals linked to positive health outcomes.

Benefits That Can't Be "Beat"

Loaded with protein, fiber, vitamins (folic acid, niacin, vitamin E, and vitamin B6), minerals (copper, magnesium, and potassium), and unsaturated fat, nuts are a powerhouse food that promote heart health. Additionally, nuts have high contents of bioactive compounds such as polyphenols, which further enhance their positive heart-health effects. Studies demonstrate that nuts reduce blood lipid concentrations and decrease blood pressure. Research has also shown that consuming nuts more than five times per week was associated with reduced incidence of heart disease. Interestingly, a review of the science on nuts shows that the proven health benefits are not specific to one kind of nut, which therefore emphasizes the importance of consuming a variety of nuts for a healthy cardiovascular system.

Eat Your Heart Out

Research suggests that eating 1½ ounces of most nuts per day as part of a low-saturated-fat diet may reduce the risk of heart disease. Luckily, there are plenty of nuts to choose from to get these health benefits, including almonds, hazelnuts, walnuts, pistachios, pine nuts, cashews, pecans, macadamia nuts, and Brazil nuts.

Taking These Recommendations to "Heart"

Of course, this is not an exhaustive list of the foods that have associated heart healthy benefits. There are a variety of foods that can have a positive effect on your cardiovascular health, and I encourage you to use additional resources such as the American Heart Association, the Mayo Clinic, and USDA MyPlate to explore the types of food that can fit into a heart-healthy diet that's right for your taste, preference, budget, and lifestyle. As always, if you have questions about certain foods or how to eat for certain medical conditions, please consult an experienced healthcare professional such as a registered dietitian.

YOGALOSOPHY
FOR INNER STRENGTH
DAILY ROUTINES

How to Approach This Program

There is no set formula for healing from loss. We each heal in our own way and at our own pace. As always, you can pick and choose what works for you; there is nothing here that you're required to do during this twelve-week journey. Note, however, that the routine I've assigned for each day is based on the planetary energy of the day of the week. In other words, you might find that sticking to the program as designed will prove to be your most beneficial course. Regardless of what you choose, plan to set aside thirty to sixty minutes per day for your physical practice.

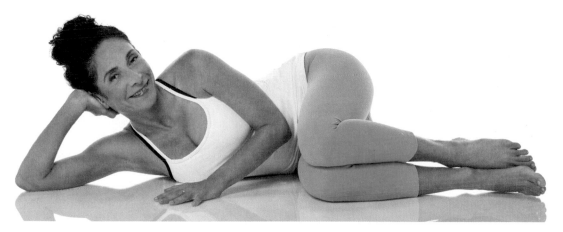

SUNDAY

BE HAPPY YOGA: I developed this routine to open the heart, awaken the spine, and release any pent-up grief or resistance. Plus, Sunday is a sun day! So it's the day to feel the joy of being the center of everything, and to shine brightly. So I incorporated cardiovascular flow yoga, which includes Sun Salutations, as well as postures to open your heart and keep your spine flexible—plus breath work to uplift you.

MONDAY

BACK-TO-BASICS YOGA: This is a basic routine designed to restore the nervous system and energize, strengthen, and stretch the body. Monday is moon-ruled, so your emotions and how you care for your body are highlighted with yoga basics. These postures will make room for your feeling and nurturing side.

TUESDAY

CARDIO MOVEMENT: This is simply a cardio workout in accordance with the theme of the week, such as running, jumping, Spinning, swimming, or dancing. Heart-rate training helps you burn fat as fuel, regulates your blood pressure and your resting heart rate, encourages blood flow, and is a natural antidepressant. Tuesday, being a Mars day, is action oriented. Mars is the go-getter, and it aims to conquer. It also rules desire and anger, so cardio work will offset excess angst by channeling that energy into physical activity.

WEDNESDAY

BOUNCE BACK! YOGA: This routine incorporates a rebounder (a mini trampoline), and provides interval training using cardio and yoga. Wednesday corresponds with the planet Mercury, which needs the mind to be engaged in multiple activities, so Wednesday is the perfect day for a variety of interval training with a mini trampoline and yoga.

THURSDAY

DAY OFF: Your body actually strengthens when you rest. A rest day is the body's opportunity to rebuild itself. Plus, sometimes it is important to sit in the emptiness and simply feel. Thursday is an expansive Jupiter day, so it's a great day to take off and expand into the world without restriction.

FRIDAY

LET GO YOGA: A sweet way to end the week, this Yin yoga routine will help you unwind by focusing on loving your body with slow stretching. You will release tension and emotions that have been stored in the tendons and fascia. Friday is Venus-ruled, so it's perfect for a sweet and gentle routine to help you let go.

SATURDAY

GET STRONG YOGALOSOPHY: This is a hybrid of my signature Yogalosophy routine, enhanced with weights for strengthening and weight-bearing resistance. Saturday is ruled by Saturn, the planet of lessons and of grounding into reality. So it's a perfect time to strengthen your bones and muscles!

SUNDAY

Be Happy Yoga Routine

You are the sun of your own universe! This day revolves around you and your happiness. Deep down, what we all want is to feel happy, but sometimes it's hard to see the pathway to elation. Let me tell you one simple route: being present in your body. This routine is designed to improve your lung capacity and infuse your blood with oxygen. It includes movements (like backbends) that open your chest and heart. It also detoxifies the body while enlivening the spine. This yoga routine is meant to give you a sense of play and joy, the perfect Sunday pick-me-up.

BREATH OF JOY!

This is a complex breathing exercise. But don't let that intimidate you! Remember to have fun. Although it may seem like a lot to coordinate, beginner's luck and playfulness go a long way, especially when it comes to being joyful. With a little practice, you'll be surprised at how intuitive this movement will become. Yoga marries the breath to the movement, so putting the two together is what makes this yoga!

Part 1: The Breathing Pattern

Practice this while standing, with your feet slightly wider than hip-width apart and knees slightly bent, so you feel grounded. Take 3 sharp sips of breath in through your nose with your mouth closed. Then open your mouth and force the exhale out of your mouth. Repeat this 3–5 times, or until the pattern becomes second nature.

Part 2: The Body Movement

From a wide stance with your knees slightly softened, swing your arms up over your head, then fling them out to the side, then back over head (just like a conductor conducting a symphony). Then let your body swing down into a forward bend and back up.

Part 3: Let's Put It All Together!

- The movement: arms up; the breath: a sharp sip in through the nose.
- Arms out to the side with a sharp sip in through the nose.
- Arms up again, another sharp sip in through the nose.
- Body swings down. Exhale out the mouth.
- Swing back up (with momentum) and inhale, continuing to the next set.

In, arms up. In, arms side. In, arms up. Exhale out the mouth, swoop down and up. Inhale.

Try this several times to get into a rhythm and then continue 5 times. Feel incredibly energized and joyful!

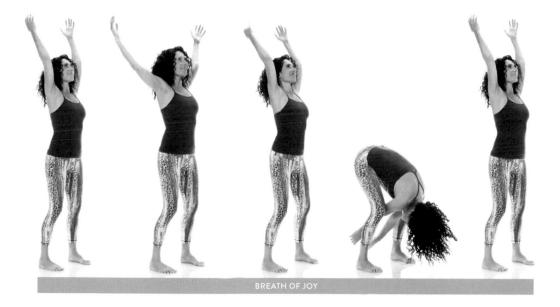

BREATH OF JOY

ARM SWING

This movement loosens and lubricates your spine.

Begin in a wide stance with softly bent knees. Swing your arms and let them flop around just like a rag doll, patting your body front and back. Swing them back and forth like a little kid on a playground. Being childlike will increase your happiness quotient. Continue for up to 2 minutes.

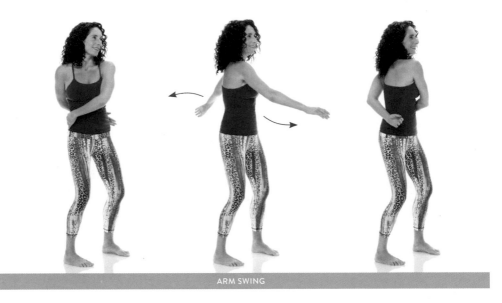

ARM SWING

HALF SALUTE/SUN BREATH (5X)

This *vinyasa* will circulate all the health, nutrients, and life force energy throughout your body.

- Begin in Mountain Pose, standing at the top of your mat with feet together.
- As you inhale, reach your arms up over your head and gaze upward.
- Exhale and firm your thighs as you fold down with a flat spine into a forward bend.
- Inhale, and bring palms up to your shins, lengthening your flat spine.

- Fold down to a forward bend and exhale all the tension out.

- Inhale to rise as you press down through the soles of your feet and swoop your arms up.

- Bring your palms back down to prayer position at your heart.

- Repeat this series 5 times.

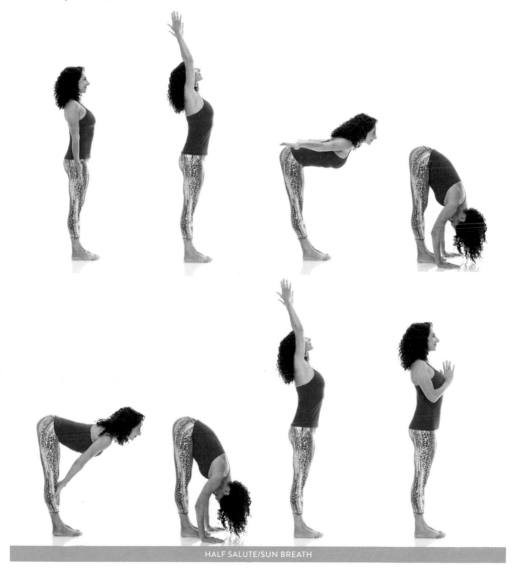

HALF SALUTE/SUN BREATH

Yoga helps reduce stress, in part, through your breathing. Breath calms your nervous system, which relaxes you, reduces any tension you may be holding, and makes you feel calm. Marrying the breath to the movement is called *vinyasa*. This is one reason why your energy feels so good when you get into a good flow.

SUN SALUTATIONS, "A" SERIES (2X)

Begin with the same Sun Breath action—only this time, after you fold forward, place your palms on the mat and step to Plank Pose.

- Stand in Mountain Pose.

- Inhale, arms up, gaze up.

- Exhale, fold down with a flat spine.

- Inhale, lengthen your spine, hands to shins.

- On the next exhale, place your palms on the mat and step your feet back for Plank Pose. Palms are aligned directly below your shoulders, and your hips, shoulders, and heels should be in a straight line. Activate your abdominals.

- Gazing forward, lower yourself down, making sure that your shoulders are no lower than your elbows as you graze your ribs/side with your elbows into Low Plank Pose.

- On an inhale, roll over your toes into Upward-Facing Dog. Keep legs straight and thighs lifted off the mat as you press the tops of the feet down into the mat.

- Roll over your toes and move back into Downward-Facing Dog. Place your palms down by your feet and step your feet back, hip-width apart (or wider if you have tight hamstrings). Push your hips back up to an apex, as if you are an inverted "V." Press your palms into the mat, especially the mound under the pointer finger. Press your chest towards your thighs. Downward-Facing Dog relaxes your nervous system, plus it lengthens and stretches the entire back of your body. Enjoy being here. Hold for 5 breaths.

- Gazing forward, lightly step or hop your feet up to your hands.

- Lift your chest and bring your palms to the shins on your inhale.

- Exhale into a Forward Bend.

- Inhale while floating back up into standing.

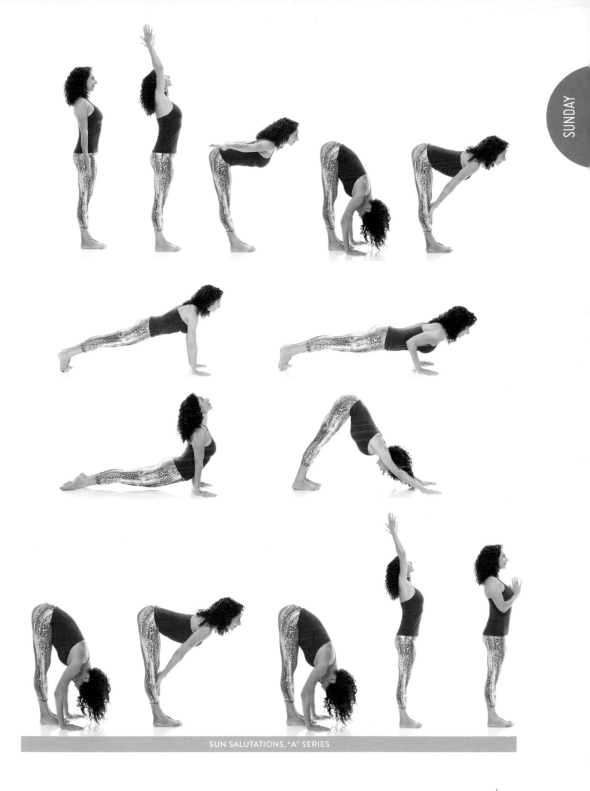

SUN SALUTATIONS, "A" SERIES

This "B" Series adds Chair Pose and Crescent Pose. Continue linking your breath to your movements and try 6 Sun Salutations with this variation.

- Start in a Mountain Pose.

- This time, as you inhale, sit down into Chair Pose. With feet together or hip-width apart, extend your arms by your ears, palms facing inward. Lower your hips down into an imaginary chair.

- Exhale, fold forward.

- Inhale, lift the heart.

- Exhale, step to Plank Pose. Inhale.

- Exhale, down to Low Plank Pose.

- Upward-Facing Dog on an inhale.

- Push back to Downward-Facing Dog.

- This time, instead of jumping back up to your hands from Downward-Facing Dog, step your right foot forward into a lunge, with knee bent at a 90° angle and your back (left) heel lifted. Then swoop your arms up into Crescent Pose. Inhale.

- Exhale, bring your hands to the floor and step back to Plank Pose. Inhale.

- Exhale, lowering down to Low Plank Pose.

- Inhale, moving to Upward-Facing Dog.

- Exhale, back to Downward-Facing Dog.

- Then repeat Crescent, now on the left side. Inhale.

- Exhale, hands to the floor, step to Plank Pose. Inhale.

- Exhale, Low Plank.

- Inhale, Upward-Facing Dog.

- Exhale, Downward-Facing Dog.

- Jump both feet to your hands, sweep your arms overhead and sink down into Chair Pose.

- Press to standing, palms together in prayer position.

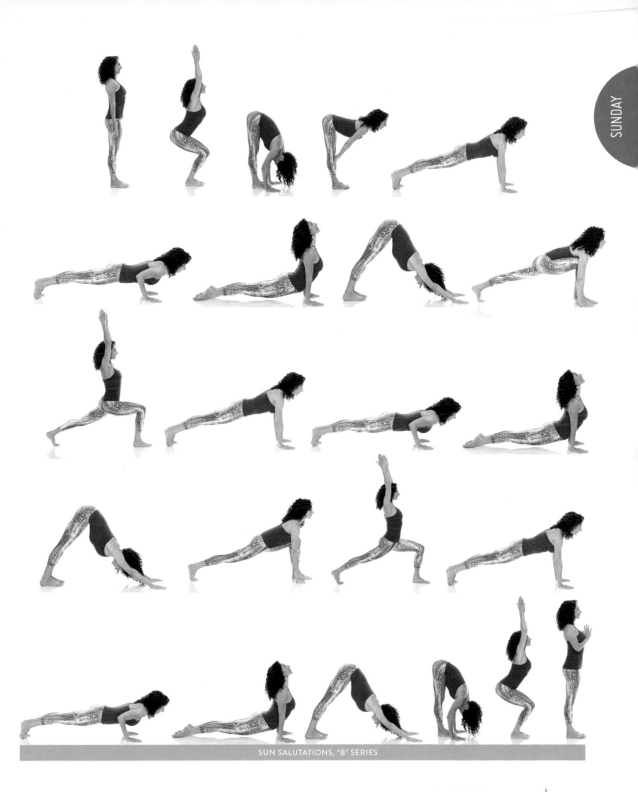

SUN SALUTATIONS, "B" SERIES

CRESCENT POSE

The lungs are related to grief and sadness. When you breathe into your lungs deeply, you begin to clear that suppressed grief. Allow yourself to feel. In order to really feel the joy, you sometimes have other feelings to process and clear.

Step your right foot between your hands and come back into a high lunge, making sure your front knee is at a 90° angle and your back leg is straight. Raise your torso to an upright position. Your feet should be hip-width apart with the back heel lifted. You may bend your back knee slightly if this is too strenuous on your hip flexors. Clasp your hands behind your back this time and open up your lungs. Take 5 breaths here.

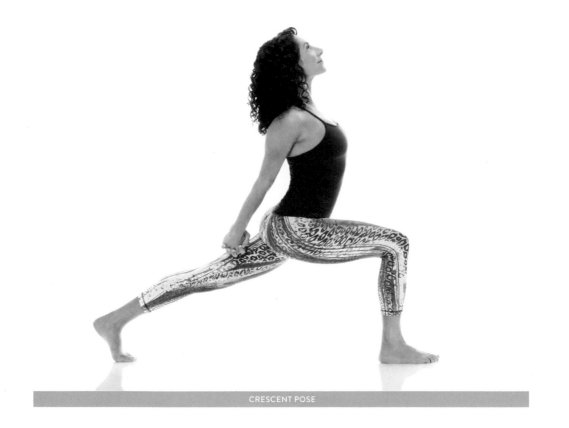

CRESCENT POSE

WARRIOR 2 POSE

In Warrior 2 Pose, as you are considering your happiness, here's a good question to ask yourself: "Is being in conflict going to make me happy today?" No. So reverse that warrior and move away from conflict. If someone or something comes at you today, you're just going to let that other person be right.

- Windmill the arms open for Warrior 2, arms extended at shoulder level with palms facing down.

- Spin your back (left) heel in flat and align your front (right) heel with your back (left) arch. Front knee remains bent at a 90° angle and torso is open to the (left) side.

- Firm your back leg.

- Feel the energy and aliveness of opposing forces. Lift up *and* sink down.

- Press your shoulders down *as* you extend energy out through your front and back fingertips.

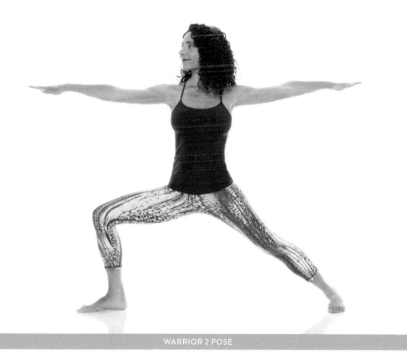

WARRIOR 2 POSE

REVERSE WARRIOR POSE

- From Warrior 2 Pose, flip your front palm and reach up and back over your head, as you allow your back (left) hand to rest lightly on the back leg.

- Spiral your chest open to the sky.

- Take 5 breaths.

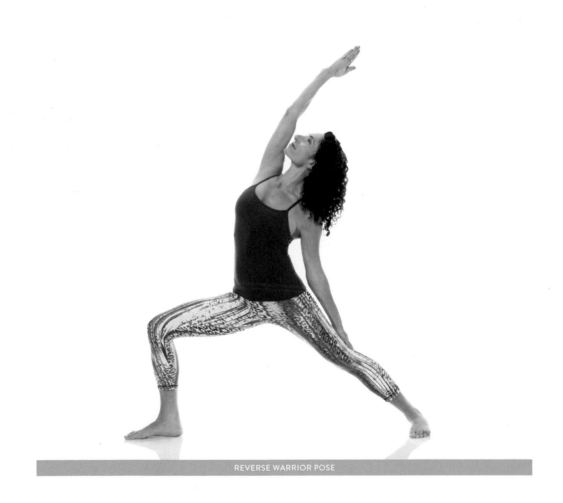

REVERSE WARRIOR POSE

TWISTING LUNGE

From Reverse Warrior Pose, cartwheel your arms down to the floor, place your left palm below your left shoulder, and reach your right arm up for a Twisting Lunge. Keep your hips level and hip points squared to the mat. Don't dump your weight into your left side.

Twist from your upper back, thinking of it as if it is a back bend. Press your left palm down to avoid dumping any tension into your back or shoulders. As you press down, it will lift your energy.

Loosening the spine allows everything to flow freely throughout your body. The yogis say that the key to remaining young is having a flexible spine. Youthfulness fills us with that childlike exuberance and joy. Twists are also excellent for detoxification, so release all that is keeping you from moving forward into your happiness.

TWISTING LUNGE

JUMPING LUNGES

As you unwind your twist, place both palms on the mat so that you are back to a lunge position.

This next movement will get your heart rate up. Be like a little kid. Stay light on your fingertips, raise your hips a little, and jump switch the legs.

Keep switching legs, increasing the pace as you're able, for 30 seconds. End on the other side.

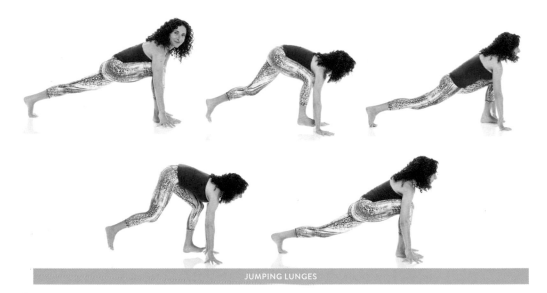

JUMPING LUNGES

SWITCH SIDES

- Crescent Pose (left side)

- Warrior 2 Pose (left side)

- Reverse Warrior Pose (left side)

- Twisting Lunge (left side)

- Jumping Lunges (30 seconds)

ROLL BACK UP TO MOUNTAIN POSE
AND DO A SUN SALUTATION

From Downward-Facing Dog, step your right foot forward.

CRESCENT POSE

Come into Crescent Pose on the right side.

TWISTING CRESCENT

From Crescent, keeping your torso upright, spinal twist to the right while extending your right arm to the right and the left arm forward. Keep both hips level and arms parallel to the floor. Hold for 5 breaths.

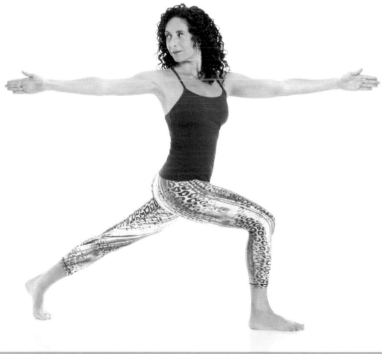

TWISTING CRESCENT

REVERSE TWISTING CRESCENT

Reach your right palm down the back straight leg and extend your left arm up and over. Hold for 5 breaths.

TWISTING LUNGE

Then sweep your left hand to the mat inside the right foot into a Twisting Lunge. Take 5 breaths.

Next step back to Plank Pose and through a *vinyasa* (Plank, Low Plank, Upward-Facing Dog, Downward-Facing Dog).

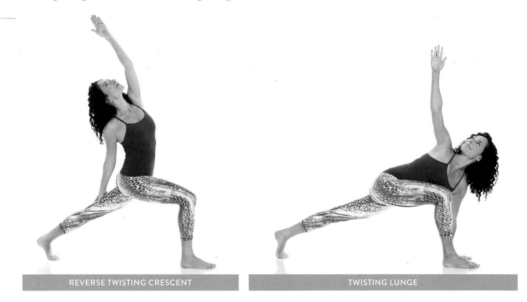

REVERSE TWISTING CRESCENT   TWISTING LUNGE

SWITCH SIDES

- Crescent Pose (left side)
- Twisting Crescent (left side)
- Reverse Twisting Crescent (left side)
- Twisting Lunge (left side)

When you're done, come to standing. High-five yourself. You're doing a great job!

EASY POSE

Sit in a cross-legged position. Take a moment t
close your eyes and place your hands on your hea
and have a moment of gratitude for your body
Think of one thing you love about your body.

Gratitude expands your happiness. Happines
is 40 percent intentional. So you are doing wha
you can today to set up intentional action towar
your well-being.

When you change your mind, you chang
how you feel. Have a great day.

SUNDAY'S PLAYLIST: Get Happy

Get happy with yoga. Bathe yourself in this *love* playlist to lift your spirits!

"Lovely Day" by Bill Withers

"Damn, I Wish I Was Your Lover" by Sophie B. Hawkins

"Feelin' Love" by Paula Cole

"Where Is the Love?" by Black Eyed Peas

"Love and Happiness" by Al Green

"Lover Lay Down" by Dave Matthews Band

"Love and Affection" by Joan Armatrading

"Storm of Prayers" by Craig Kohland & Shaman's Dream

MONDAY

Basics Yoga Routine

40-50
MINUTES

...a practice are good for anyone, they're particularly good when experiencing heartbreak and loss. Yoga will bring you emotional balance, calm your mind, and strengthen your physical body.

Yoga not only balances your physical body, it realigns your subtle body as well. The subtle body consists of your energy body and your chakras—as well as many tiny points all throughout your system that, once opened, will allow your energy to flow more easily, thus giving you more access to your life force.

Monday's practice relates to the Moon and how you feel. Be open to noticing how you feel, and feel your way through the routine, carefully selecting what works and leaving the rest behind.

Feel free to begin with Sun Salutations (page 36) before moving into this standing sequence.

UJJAYI BREATHING

Practice *ujjayi* (*oo-jai*) breathing during yoga. *Ujjayi* translates as "victorious breath" and is also commonly called "ocean breath" due to the sound it creates when done correctly. This breathing will become second nature over time, so be patient with yourself as you explore. Here's how to do it:

Low Lunge

- Step your right foot forward between your hands.

- Keep your hands and your back knee on your mat. If you want a deeper stretch, keep your front knee aligned over heel and either place both hands on your front (right) thigh or reach both arms up.

- If you like, activate your hip stretch by slightly scooping your tailbone under and finding extension in the upper body.

- After 3 breaths, bring your hands back down to the floor.

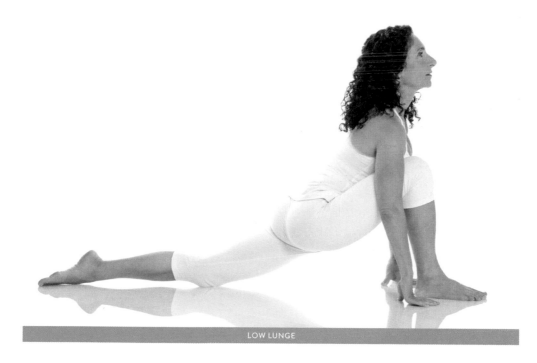

LOW LUNGE

Hamstring Stretch

- With hands on either side of your foot, shove your hips back and straighten your right leg, extending out through a flexed heel.

- Lengthen your spine by reaching your sternum toward the top of your foot.

- Take 3 deep breaths.

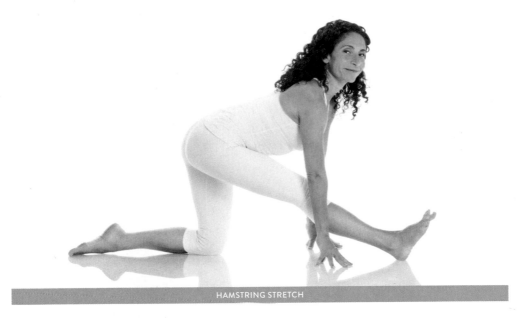

HAMSTRING STRETCH

SWITCH SIDES

Bend your knee and transition through Downward-Facing Dog. Step your left foot forward to repeat on the left side, then find your way back to Downward Dog.

- Lunge (left side)

- Hamstring Stretch (left side)

Plank Pose

- Shift your weight forward so that your body is straight and your weight is balanced evenly between your palms below the shoulders and feet hip-width apart.

- Draw in your navel and firm your thighs.

- Your hips should be aligned with your shoulders. The back has a tendency to sag and sway or sometimes hips lift up, so find a straight body position, literally like a plank. Engage your abdominals. It also helps to push into the mat with your palms so as not to dump tension into your shoulders.

- Take 3 deep breaths. Then, with control, lower to your belly.

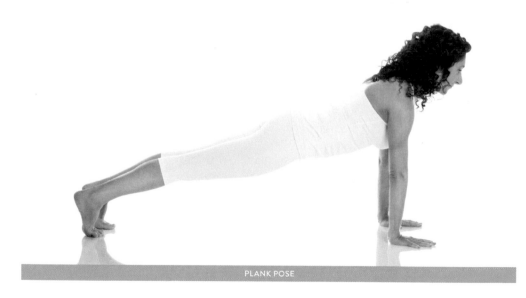

PLANK POSE

Cobra Pose

- Position your palms with your thumbs directly below your shoulders.

- Hug your elbows in toward your side body.

- Make your thighs firm. Press the instep sides of your feet together with the tops of your feet pressing actively into the mat.

- Lift your chest off the mat and gaze forward.

- Lift the palms off the mat for a moment and then place your palms back down as you raise your chest a bit higher with elbows in and shoulders back. Take 3 deep breaths then lower your chest.

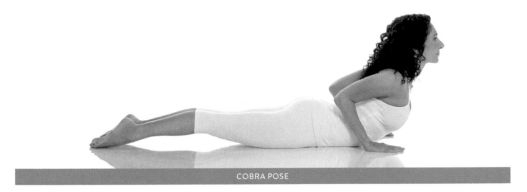

COBRA POSE

Child's Pose

- Press your hips back to your heels and bow down, your active arms extended out in front of you.

- Let your knees either open or close and allow your forehead and the tip of your nose to rest on your mat.

- Take 3 slow deep breaths.

- Tuck your toes under and press your hips up to Downward-Facing Dog.

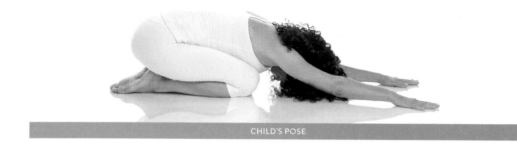

CHILD'S POSE

VINYASA (3X)

Match the breath to the movement. Repeat each move 3 times with 1 breath on each move.

- Inhale—Plank Pose.

- Exhale—Low Plank Pose.

- Inhale—Cobra Pose.

- Exhale—Downward-Facing Dog.

After 3 sets, walk your feet to your hands and roll up to standing, one vertebra at a time.

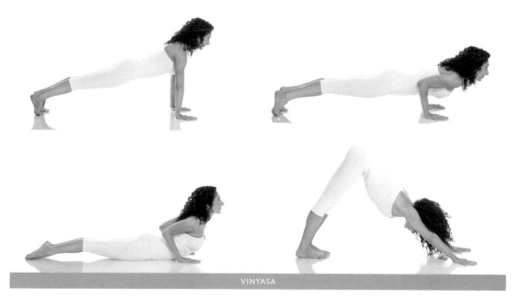

VINYASA

SUN SALUTATIONS (3X)

See Sunday's routine for more detailed instructions (page 36).

- Begin standing in Mountain Pose.

- Inhale—Arms swoop up.

- Exhale—Hinge at hips: Forward Fold.

- Inhale—Flat back, lift chest.

- Exhale—Palms to floor, step back to Plank Pose.

- Inhale—Top of Plank Pose.

- Exhale—Low Plank Pose.

- Inhale—Cobra Pose. *Option to replace Cobra with Upward-Facing Dog.*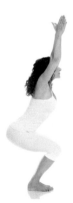

- Exhale—Downward-Facing Dog.

- Inhale—Step feet forward.

- Exhale—Forward Bend.

- Inhale—Lift chest.

- Exhale—Fold.

- Inhale—Float back to standing, arms overhead. *Option to replace with Chair Pose. Arms swoop up, hips sink down.*

- Exhale—Arms down, Mountain Pose.

Repeat the Sun Salute two more times.

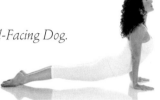

Twisting Lunge

- Step back into a runner's lunge on your right side, and place your left palm on the floor below your shoulder.

- Extend your right arm up to the ceiling so that you are in a twist.

- On each inhale, lengthen your spine; on each exhale, twist from your middle a little deeper.

- After 3 deep breaths, place the hands on either side of your foot and move through a *vinyasa* to repeat the sequence on the left side.

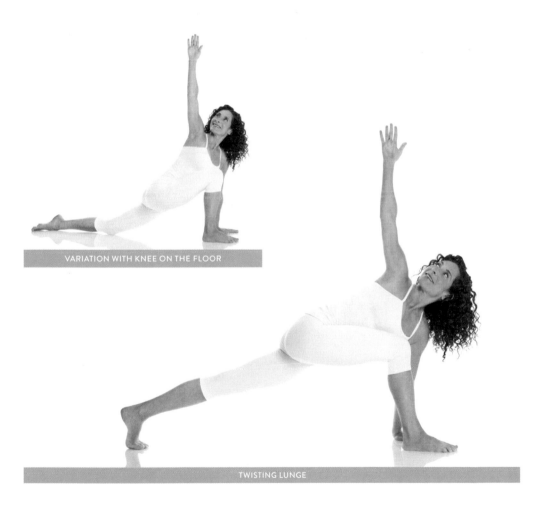

VARIATION WITH KNEE ON THE FLOOR

TWISTING LUNGE

SWITCH SIDES

- Vinyasa (Plank Pose, Low Plank Pose, Upward-Facing Dog, Downward-Facing Dog)
- Crescent Pose/Diagonal Pose (left side)
- Warrior 3 (standing on left leg)
- Extended Leg Pose (standing on left leg)
- Tree Pose (standing on left leg)
- Twisting Lunge (left side)
- Step back to Plank

ARMS/ABS

Plank Pose

Hold Plank Pose for 30–60 seconds. Build up each week by adding 30 seconds. Challenge yourself by raising the right toes and then the left toes off the mat for 15 seconds.

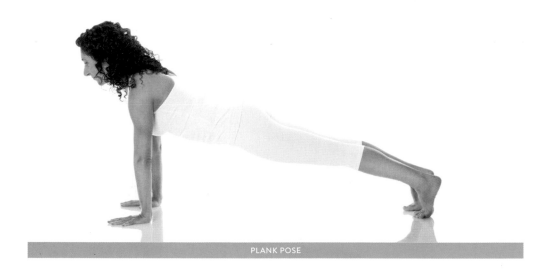

PLANK POSE

Side Plank

- From Plank, walk your right palm in to the center of your mat beneath your face.
- Stack or stagger your feet and flex them as you rock your body weight onto the right hand and onto the outer edge of the right foot.
- Press your right palm into the mat and lift the underside of your waist up.
- Align your shoulders, head, hips, and heels.
- Take 3 deep breaths.
- EXTRA CHALLENGE: Raise your top leg up.
- Come through Plank and switch sides to do the Side Plank on the left side.

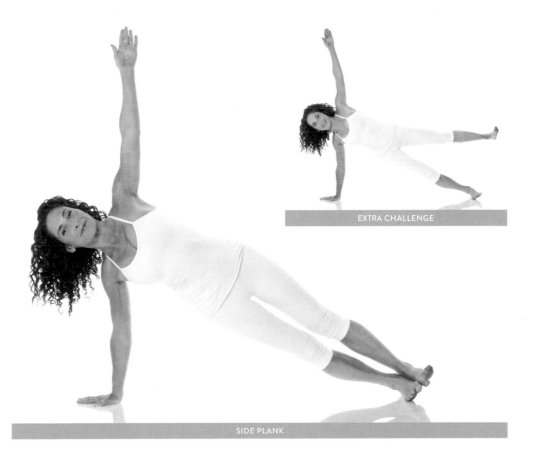

EXTRA CHALLENGE

SIDE PLANK

Forearm Plank

- From Plank, bring your forearms to the mat, parallel to each other. Align your elbows below your shoulders.

- Keep your hips level with your shoulders. Firm your thighs and hold.

- Engage your abdominals as you push into the mat and activate your muscles.

- Breathe and hold here for 30 seconds. For endurance and strength, build up by adding 30 seconds each week.

- Lower your torso and legs to the mat.

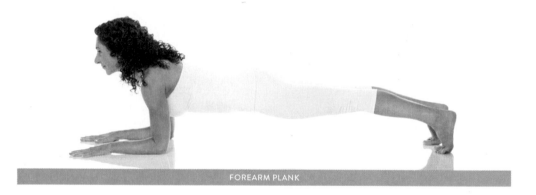

FOREARM PLANK

Sphinx Pose

- Keep your forearms in Forearm Plank alignment.

- Press forearms down as you lift your chest up and extend your sternum to the sky.

- Press your hip bones into the floor and slightly scoop the tailbone, pressing the pubic bone into the mat as if you could lengthen your spine and lower back.

- Take 5 deep breaths.

- Lower your head down and rest it to one side.

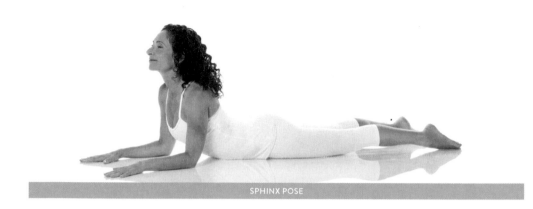

SPHINX POSE

Locust Pose

- From your belly, look straight ahead and reach your arms behind you, clasping your hands behind your back.

- Take a deep breath in and lift as much of your upper and lower body off the mat as you can. Squeeze your legs together.

- Take 5 breaths and lower your head; unclasp your hands and rest your head to the other side for 30 seconds.

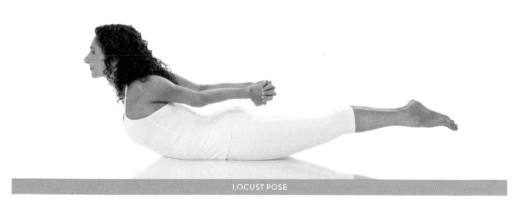

LOCUST POSE

Child's Pose

Hold Child's Pose for 5 breaths.

Downward-Facing Dog

From Child's Pose, press back to Downward-Facing Dog.

Extend to Three-Legged Dog

Extend the right leg back into Three-Legged Dog, moving into some abdominal work.

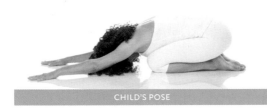

CHILD'S POSE

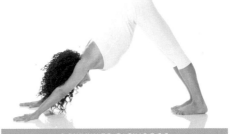

DOWNWARD-FACING DOG

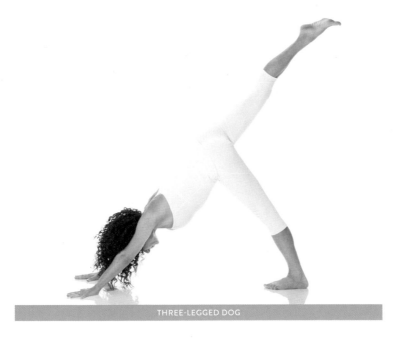

THREE-LEGGED DOG

Knee-In to Three-Legged Dog (8x)

- From Three-Legged Dog, exhale and shift the body weight forward into your hands as you draw the right knee in toward your forehead.

- Inhale, pressing back and extending the right leg back to Three-Legged Dog.

- Do this 8 times. Then switch to the left leg for another 8 times.

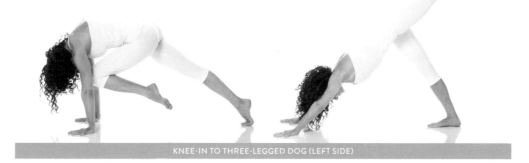

KNEE-IN TO THREE-LEGGED DOG (RIGHT SIDE)

SWITCH SIDES

- Do Knee-In to Three-Legged Dog 8 times on the left side.

- Return to Downward Dog. From there, lower down and find your way to sitting.

KNEE-IN TO THREE-LEGGED DOG (LEFT SIDE)

Boat Pose (3x)

- Sit up on your sit bones and press your lower back/kidney area forward.

- Grab behind your hamstrings and use the leverage to lift your chest up toward the ceiling, straightening your spine. Soften your ribs closed and engage your belly.

- Lift your feet and raise them up in alignment with your knees.

- Release the arms. Extend them forward at shoulder height, with palms facing in.

- Then try to straighten your legs.

- Hold for 30 seconds. You may add a breath to this each week to build on the pose.

- If you need extra support, place your hands on the floor behind you. Repeat 3 times.

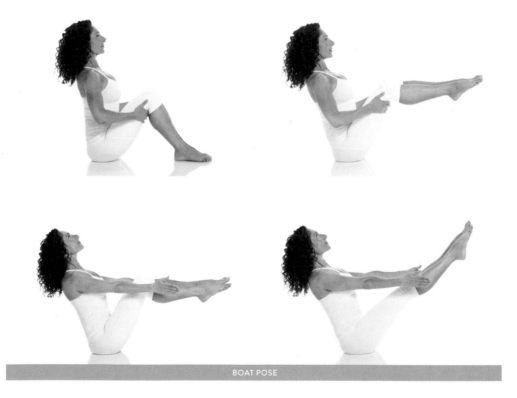

BOAT POSE

Cobbler's Pose

- From sitting, fan your knees open to the sides and bring the soles of your feet together

- On an inhale, grip your feet and lengthen your spine. As you exhale, fold forward.

- Hold the pose for 5–10 breaths.

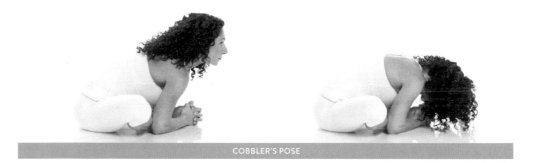

COBBLER'S POSE

One-Legged Forward Bend

- Keep your right leg bent and extend your left leg straight out in front of you.

- Take a deep inhale and lengthen your spine; on your exhale, fold forward.

- Hold for 5–10 breaths. Then rise up to sitting.

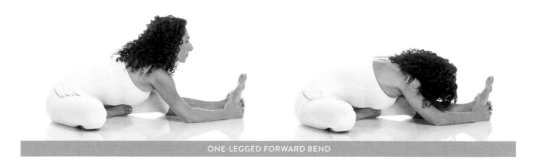

ONE-LEGGED FORWARD BEND

Pigeon Pose

- Keep your right knee bent and lean to the right as you swing your left leg behind you.
- Your right knee should be open to the side, on the outside of your right shoulder, with the foot aiming toward the left hip bone. Your hips should be squared to the mat.
- Bring your hands in front of your shin and then slowly lower down.
- Keep your right foot flexed to protect and maintain the integrity of the knee.
- Hold this pose for up to 2 minutes.
- Rise and find your way out of the pose just as you found your way into it.
- Jiggle the legs and switch to the left side.

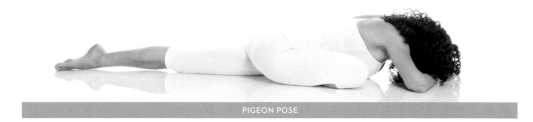

PIGEON POSE

SWITCH SIDES

- One-Legged Forward Bend (left side)
- Pigeon Pose (left side)

Seated Forward Bend

- Extend both legs out in front of you. Move the fleshy part of the butt to the sides. Feel how your sit bones are planted to the floor.
- Take a deep inhale and extend your arms up as you lengthen your spine. Then exhale and fold forward.

- Extend your chest toward the tops of your feet to keep a flat spine. To aid you in the stretch you can wrap a strap or towel around your foot.
- After 1 minute, slowly roll up to sitting, bend your knees in, and roll onto your back.

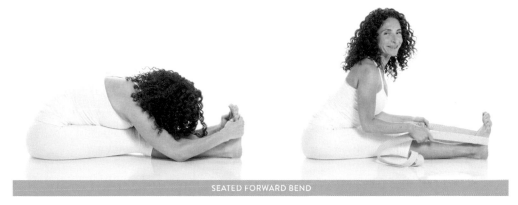

SEATED FORWARD BEND

Happy Baby Pose

- Hug your knees in to your chest and reach for the insides or outsides of your feet.
- Open your knees so they are outside your ribs on either side of your torso; aim the soles of your feet up to the ceiling.
- Keep your shoulders and upper back down on the floor. Arch your back so that more of your lower back and spine are on the floor.
- Open and breathe for 5–10 breaths.
- Release and lower your feet to your mat.

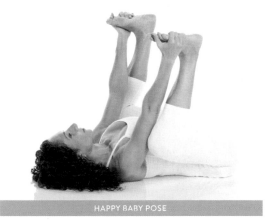

HAPPY BABY POSE

Bridge Pose (3x)

- Bend your knees with feet parallel on the mat so that you can graze your heels with your fingertips.

- On an exhale, press your feet down to raise your hips up and peel your spine off the mat with your arms down by your sides.

- Keep your knees in alignment with your hips. Engage your inner thighs.

- Lengthen your lower back by scooping the tailbone.

- Clasp your hands beneath you and wriggle up onto your shoulders, or reach your arms over your head and rest them on the floor. Modification: Place a yoga brick under your sacrum (lower spine, near your tailbone) for support.

- After 5 breaths, lower your hips (or remove brick and lower) back down to the mat. Repeat this 2 more times.

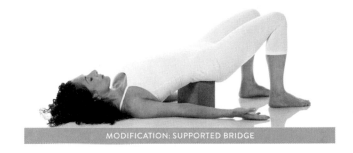

MODIFICATION: SUPPORTED BRIDGE

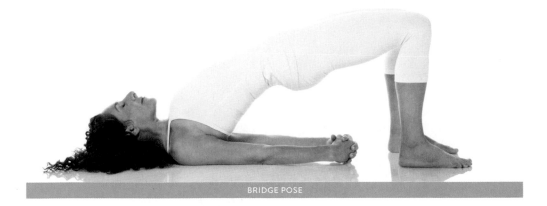

BRIDGE POSE

Reclining Twist

Note: For Reclining Twist it is more important to keep both shoulders on the mat than it is to get your knee to the floor.

- From supine position, hug both knees in and extend your arms out to your sides at shoulder level with palms facing down.

- Slowly twist your legs to the right, keeping your knees bent.

- Look to the left.

- Use your right hand to assist with your twist.

- After 5 deep breaths, bring yourself back through the center and mindfully switch sides and repeat.

- When you're done, come back through the center.

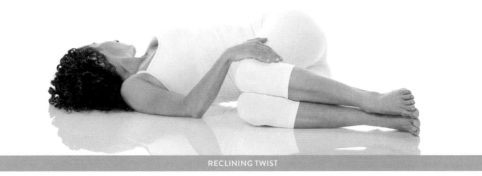

RECLINING TWIST

Shoulder Stand

- From a supine position with arms down by your sides, bend your knees and contract your abs.

- Inhale. As you exhale, bring your legs up with your knees in by pressing your arms into the floor.

- Support and lift your back as you place your palms on your lower back and draw your elbows toward each other.

- There should be very little weight on your neck. Do not move your head around.

- Walk your hands up toward your back ribs, aligning your hips with your shoulders. With this support and the knees still bent, draw your tailbone toward your pubic bone and internally rotate your thighs.

- On your next inhale, straighten your legs up toward the ceiling, extending up through the balls of the feet to lengthen and strengthen your legs. Reach up!

- Relax and breathe here for 30 seconds. Increase the length of time by 30 seconds each week until you are able to hold for up to 5 minutes.

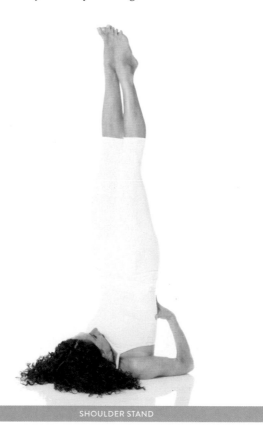

SHOULDER STAND

Deaf Man's Pose

- To move into Deaf Man's Pose, slowly bend your knees and let them drop to either side of your head if it feels okay on your neck. (If not, skip this pose and simply bring your knees to your forehead, then slowly roll your spine down one vertebrae at a time.)

- With your knees on either side of the head, near your ears, reach for your heels (if you can) and pull your knees closer in toward your shoulders.

- Hold this pose for 5 deep breaths.

- When you are ready, bring your hands to your lower back and knees to your forehead.

- Slowly, with control, keeping the knees bent, lower down one vertebra at a time.

- When your hips reach the mat, hug your knees in to your chest and rock gently from side to side.

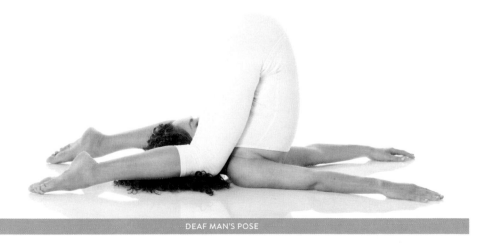

DEAF MAN'S POSE

SAVASANA/CORPSE POSE

- Lie with your legs outstretched and slightly apart and your feet flopping open. Relax your shoulders down, away from your ears. Get as comfortable as you can.

- Flip your palms upward. Be receptive and relaxed.

Enjoy this feeling of your body, after having been touched, moved, and loved up by you. Feel the sensation of total relaxation as you allow your body to sink down into the mat, simply allowing yourself to surrender completely.

All is well. You are exactly where you are supposed to be. Taking the time for yourself like this is both an act of self-love and an act of faith. It is enough to be right here, in this moment, just as you are.

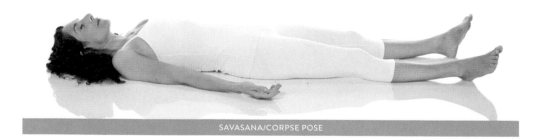

SAVASANA/CORPSE POSE

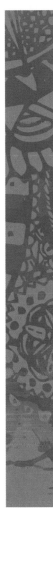

MONDAY'S PLAYLIST: Back-to-Basics

This mellow and uplifting mix is one of my favorites to play when I work with my clients.

"Night Bird" by Deep Forest

"Everloving" by Moby

"Teardrop" by Massive Attack

"The Glass Bead Game" by Thievery Corporation

"#41" by Dave Matthews Band

"Tarana" by Thievery Corporation featuring Ustad Sultan Khan

"Slow Marimbas" by Peter Gabriel

"Distractions" by Zero 7

"I Still Care for You" by Ray LaMontagne

"Higher Ground" by Weekend Players

"Even After All" by Finley Quaye

"River" by Leon Bridges

"Ziricote" by Coyote Oldman

TUESDAY

Cardio Movement

Cardio day. Let's not forget that in order to take care of our emotional heart we must reflect that in the actions of the physical heart. Getting your heart rate up and doing cardiovascular work will help to lift your spirits as well as condition your heart against disease. One of the best things you can do for grief is a heart-pumping workout. For the next twelve weeks, I will suggest a weekly cardio activity. Feel free to branch off on your own and get your heart rate up in a way that suits you, and add cardio on additional days if you feel inspired.

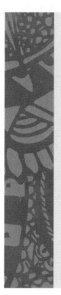

TUESDAY'S PLAYLIST: Cardio Mix

I made this mix in the good old days of being a Spinning instructor. If you want to follow suit and spin to this, here's a routine:

1. Warm up

2. Standing walking

3. Hands to 3 and push through resistance on chorus

4. Side to side, back and front

5. Climb seated

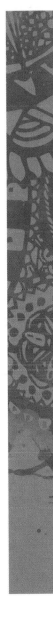

6. Sprint in saddle

7. Jumps in and out of saddle

8. Strong jog with resistance building

9. In-and-out-of-saddle rhythmic climb

10. Sprints out of saddle on chorus

11. Trot home

Otherwise, just enjoy the cardio of your choice!

"Woody & Dutch on the Slow Train to Peking" by Rickie Lee Jones

"Magalenha" by Sérgio Mendes featuring Carlinhos Brown

"Spill the Wine" by War

"Lonesome Day" by Bruce Springsteen

"Grandma's Hands" by Bill Withers

"Someday" by The Strokes

"Boogie on Reggae Woman" by Stevie Wonder

"In My Place" by Coldplay

"Sleepy Maggie" by Ashley MacIsaac

"Semi-Charmed Life" by Third Eye Blind

"Peace Train" by Cat Stevens

WEDNESDAY
Bounce Back! Yoga Routine

40–50
MINUTES

A rebounder is a mini trampoline that can be easily stored at home. It's a perfect way to get your heart rate up while being easy on your joints. No shoes required! It's excellent for your lymphatic system, for toning, and for cardiovascular conditioning. Most important, it will increase your joy . . . as bouncing tends to do. I like to think of this routine as rebounding from your heartbreak and bouncing back into you.

I developed this routine when I was in India on a silent meditation retreat, where I found a rusty old mini trampoline and a yoga mat. This interval training routine alternates between 5 minutes of trampoline cardio work and 5 minutes of yoga. Interval training has been proven to be very effective for short workouts, since you're essentially shocking your body into shape. I like this routine, in part because it's broken up into 5-minute sections, and in part because it trains you like an athlete for a most efficient workout.

If you don't have a trampoline, you can do the moves in your aerobic shoes just the same. Just be sure to have fun!

WARM-UP BOUNCING ON MINI TRAMPOLINE

5 minutes

Freestyle jump. The mini tramp/rebounder is so fun. It makes you feel like a kid! I like to bounce up and down and side to side, front and back. Whatever feels good, do it.

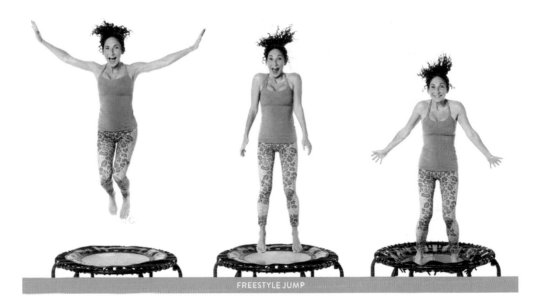

FREESTYLE JUMP

SUN SALUTATIONS, A SERIES & B SERIES

5 minutes, 3 sets of each

Continue to warm up the body and spine with 3 sets of A Salutes followed by 3 sets of B Salutes. For more detailed instructions, refer back to Sunday's Be Happy Yoga routine on page 36.

Sun Salutations, "A" Series (3x)

- Stand at the top of your mat. Get centered in Mountain Pose.
- Inhale and reach your arms up overhead, palms touching at the top.
- Exhale, hinging at your hips to forward fold.
- Inhale, lifting the heart.
- Exhale, fold, and step back to Plank.
- Inhale, move to top of Plank.
- Slowly lower down on the exhale to Low Plank Pose.
- Inhale, arching the back, to Upward-Facing Dog.
- Exhale, pressing back to Downward-Facing Dog. Take 3–5 breaths.
- Look forward and step or hop to the top of your mat.
- Inhale with a flat back.
- Exhale into a fold.
- On an inhale press up to standing.

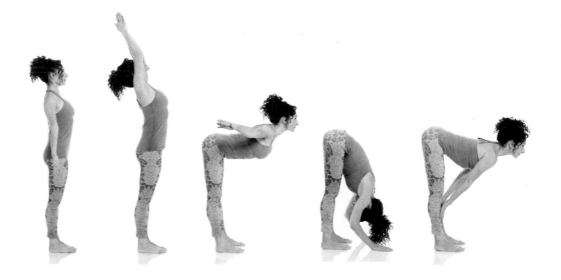

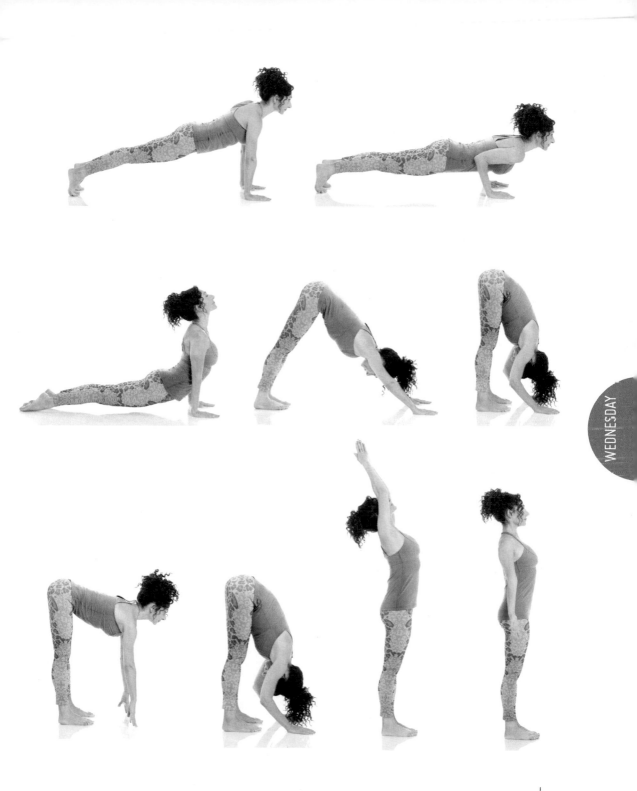

Sun Salutations, "B" Series (3x)

- Begin standing.

- Inhale and sink down into Chair Pose.

- Exhale and fold into a Forward Bend.

- Inhale while lifting the heart.

- Exhale into a Plank Pose (or jump to Low Plank Pose).

- Inhale into an Upward-Facing Dog.

- Exhale, pressing back to Downward-Facing Dog.

- On an inhale, step your right leg forward to Crescent Pose with your arms up.

- Exhale, sweep your arms down, and step back to Plank. (OPTION: keep your right toes lifted as you lower down. When you come all the way down, place your foot on the floor.)

- Inhale, arch, and lift to Upward-Facing Dog.

- Exhale into Downward-Facing Dog.

- Step your left leg forward into a Crescent on the left side. Inhale, arms up.

- On an exhale bring your palms to the mat and step back. (OPTION: keep left toes lifted.)

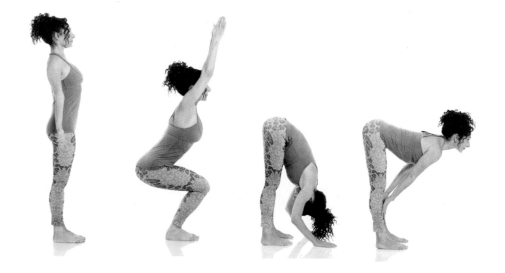

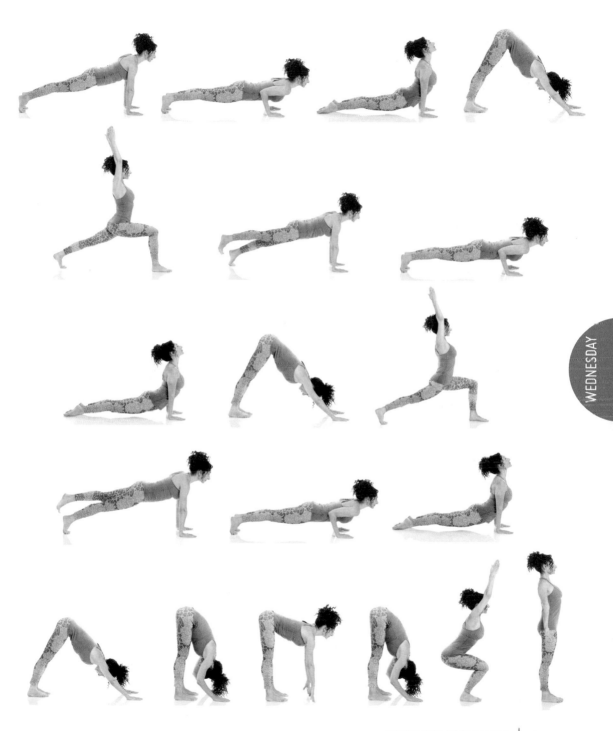

- On an inhale, arch to Upward-Facing Dog.
- Roll over your toes and press back to Downward-Facing Dog. Take 3–5 breaths.
- Look at your hands; lightly hop your feet to your hands.
- Inhale, lifting your chest.
- Exhale into a fold.
- Inhale, sweeping arms up to Chair Pose.
- Exhale, pressing to standing.
- Repeat 2 more times.

BOUNCING: SET 1

5 minutes, 1 minute per movement

Jumping Jacks

As you jump, your legs and arms should move together, one movement per bounce. On the first bounce jump your legs apart with your arms overhead; on the second bounce bring your legs back in and your arms to the sides.

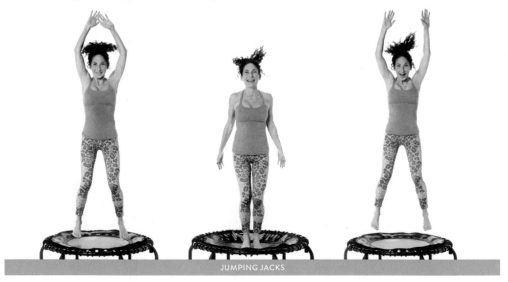

JUMPING JACKS

Cross Jacks

For the bounces when your legs are together, alternate crossing your right leg in front of your left. Then, after a bounce with your legs apart, cross your left leg in front of your right.

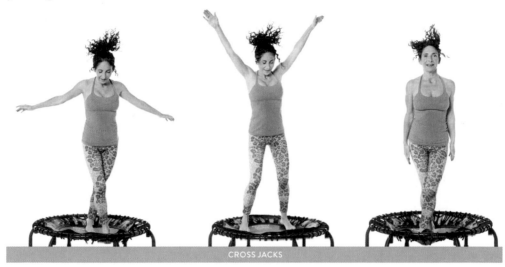

CROSS JACKS

WEDNESDAY

Right-Side Jacks

With these the variation is on the bounce when your legs are apart—only you move just your right leg out, with both feet landing together.

Left-Side Jacks

This time, move the left leg out, then land both feet together.

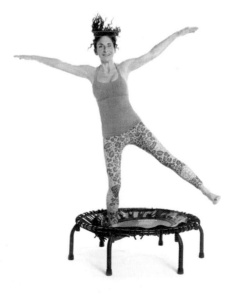

SIDE JACKS

Around-the-World Jumping Jacks

- Face front for 4 jacks

- Rotate 90° clockwise (to the right) for 4 jacks.

- Rotate another 90° clockwise for 4.

- Rotate another 90° clockwise for 4, bringing you back to the front.

- Repeat going counterclockwise (to the left).

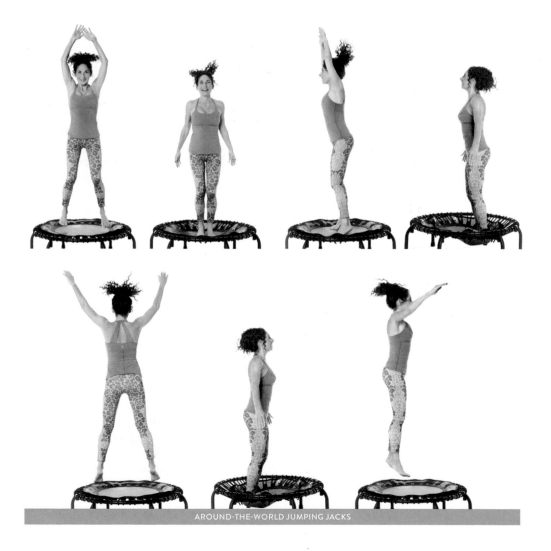

AROUND-THE-WORLD JUMPING JACKS

BOUNCING: SET 2

5 minutes, 1 minute per movement

Knee Kick-Up

Alternate bringing up one knee with each jump. So: jump and bring your right knee up; jump and bring your left knee up.

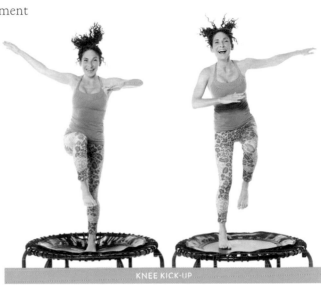

KNEE KICK-UP

Run in place, knees up

Maniac fast feet—double time!

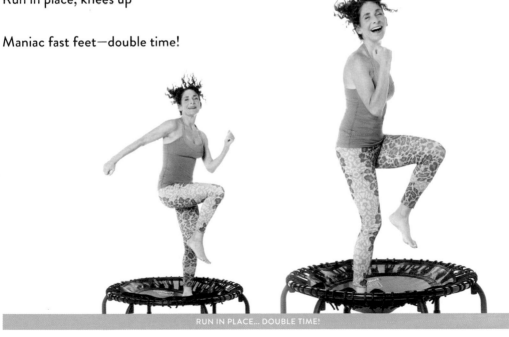

RUN IN PLACE... DOUBLE TIME!

Bounce side to side on the trampoline

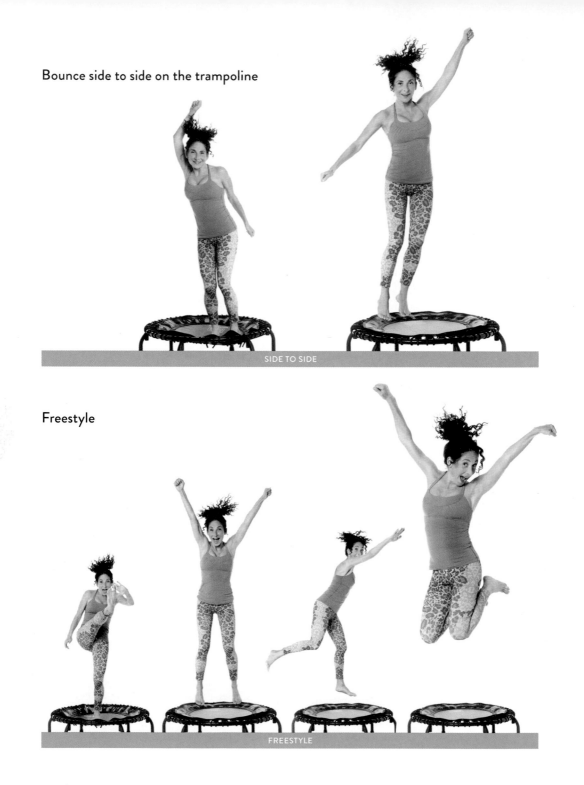

SIDE TO SIDE

Freestyle

FREESTYLE

5 minutes. Hold each balance pose for 30 seconds or for 5 deep breaths.

Tree Pose

- From Mountain Pose, shift your body weight to your right leg.
- Find a gazing point and focus on your breath to still your mind.
- Bend your left knee and open the leg out to the left, placing the so
  foot to the inside of your calf or inner right thigh.
- Reach your arms up overhead, with the option to gaze upward if
  your balance. When the gaze is still, the mind is still.

Half Chair Pose

- From Tree Pose,
  cross your left ankle
  over your right knee.
- With your arms
  continuing to extend
  upward, sink your
  hips back and down
  as if into an imagi-
  nary chair.
- Flex your foot to
  protect your knee.
- Slowly come back up
  to standing on your
  right leg.

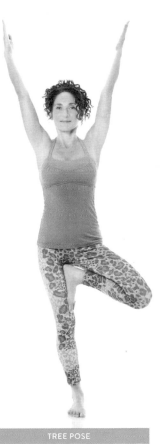

TREE POSE

e

in your gazing point as you remain balanced on your right leg.

ur left leg back as you tip your body forward. Firm your standing leg

ve into a "T" position.

y bring your arms by your hips or out to the side (airplane arms).

s

vard until your fingertips or palms are on the floor, then raise

ck leg up into a standing split.

our chest down and aim it toward the top of your foot.

ur neck.

vn with control and roll up

rtebra at a time.

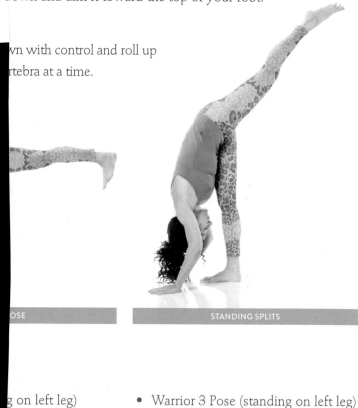

STANDING SPLITS

g on left leg)   • Warrior 3 Pose (standing on left leg)

anding on left leg)   • Standing Splits (standing on left leg)

STRENGTH

BOUNCING: SET 3

5 minutes, 1 minute per movement

Leg-Back Jack (Alternating-Leg Kick Backs)

Jump and bend your right knee, kicking your heel toward your right butt cheek. Repeat on the left side. Alternate between the two.

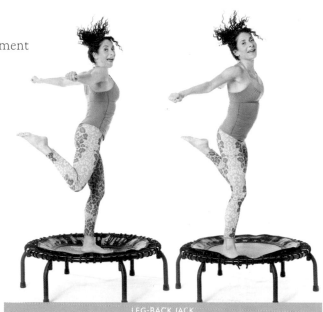

LEG-BACK JACK

Forward Kick

FORWARD KICK

WEDNESDAY

Side Kick

Twisting Mashed Potato (Double Count)

Twisting Mashed Potato (Single Count)

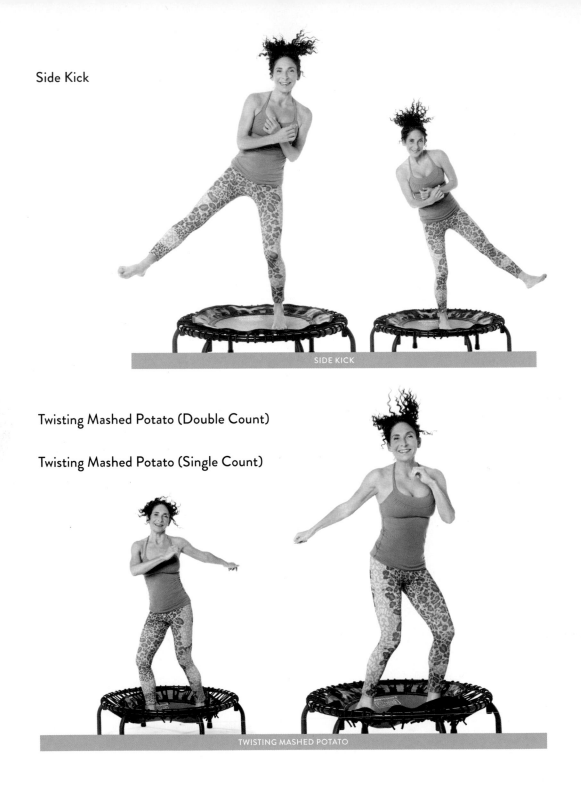

SIDE KICK

TWISTING MASHED POTATO

ABDOMINAL WORK

5 minutes, 1 minute per pose or movement

Forearm Plank

- Come to your hands and knees. then bring your forearms to the floor parallel to each other, with your elbows directly below your shoulders.
- With toes curled under, firm your thighs.
- Press down through your forearms.
- Engage your abdominals so as not to allow your back to sway. Keep hips at shoulder level.

WEDNESDAY

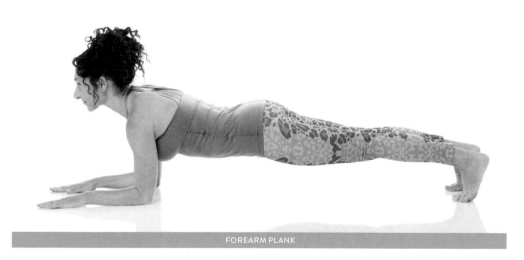

FOREARM PLANK

Legs-Straight-Up Sit-Ups

- Lie on your back and extend your legs straight up, feet directly over your hips.

- Do a sit-up reaching up for your feet.

- Repeat for 1 minute.

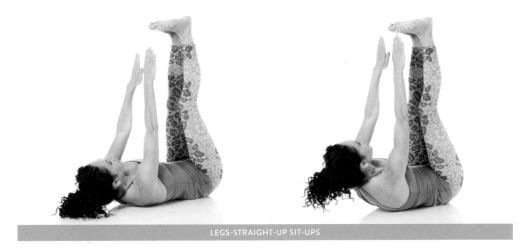

LEGS-STRAIGHT-UP SIT-UPS

Legs-Split Sit-Ups

- For these sit-ups, open your legs wide and bring your palms together.

- Reach forward and pulse up for 1 minute.

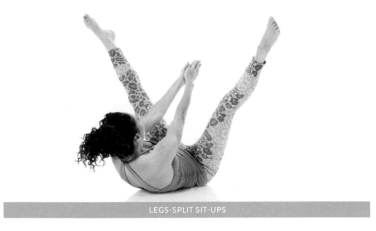

LEGS-SPLIT SIT-UPS

Scissor Legs

- With your legs still lifted in the air, close them together. Stack one hand on the other to support your lower back.

- Lift your torso to engage your abs while lowering your right leg. Then raise your right leg while lowering your left leg, scissoring your legs.

- Keep your lower back on the mat (no space should be between your lower back and the mat).

- Repeat, alternating, for 1 minute.

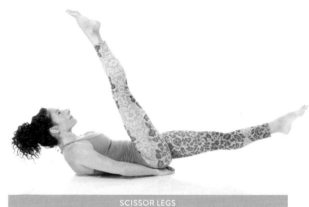

SCISSOR LEGS

Raised Knee-In

- With palms stacked under your lower back, press the small of the back into the floor.

- Extend your legs out, heels hovering 3 inches off the floor.

- Keeping your right leg hovering, bring your left knee toward your chest. Hold.

- Straighten your left leg while bringing your right knee in.

- Repeat, alternating, for 1 minute.

RAISED KNEE-IN

5 minutes, 1 minute per pose

Reclining Pigeon Pose

- Hug both knees to your chest. Then place your feet on the floor with knees bent.

- Cross your right ankle over your left knee and allow your right knee to fan open to the right. Flex your right foot.

- Thread your hands behind your left leg and gently draw your leg in for an outer hip stretch on your right side.

- Keep both shoulders on the mat. Relax. Hold for 1 minute.

RECLINING PIGEON POSE

Hamstring Stretch (Supine)

- Lower your left foot to the mat and extend your right leg with foot flexed.

- Reach behind your right hamstring and gently draw your leg closer to your torso. You may bend the right knee a little if this is too intense. Hold for 1 minute.

HAMSTRING STRETCH (SUPINE)

Reclining Twist

Draw both knees to your chest and move into your favorite twist—with your legs to the right while looking to the left.

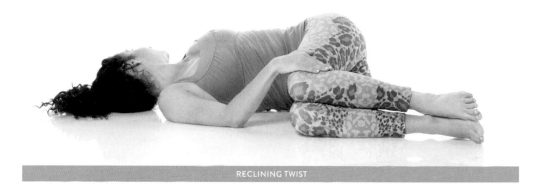

RECLINING TWIST

SWITCH SIDES

Hug your knees in and repeat all on the left side.

- Reclining Pigeon Pose (left foot crossed)

- Hamstring Stretch (left side)

- Reclining Twist (legs to the left, look to the right)

Reclining Butterfly Pose

Still lying on your back, place your feet on the floor with your knees bent. Allow your knees to fan open to the sides for an inner thigh stretch. Hold for 1 minute.

Note: You may place pillows under both sides for support. If this pose bothers your lower back at all, please skip it.

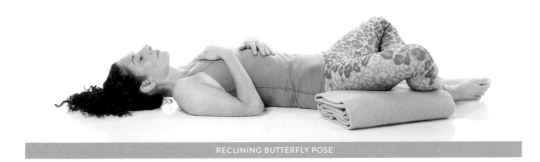

RECLINING BUTTERFLY POSE

CLOSING POSE

Wrap it up with any pose that completes the routine for you today.

SAVASANA/CORPSE POSE

Extend your legs and flip your palms upward as you allow your feet to flop open to the sides. Get as comfortable as you can and take 3 long deep breaths. Remain here for as long as you wish, allowing any extra tension to drain right out of your body. Anything that's old or holding you back is now being released.

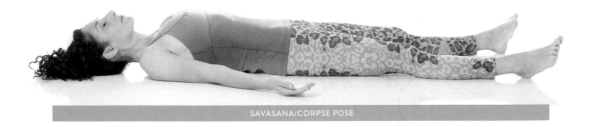

SAVASANA/CORPSE POSE

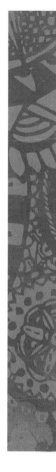

WEDNESDAY'S PLAYLIST: BOUNCE BACK

As you go through this interval routine, alternate your own favorite mellow song with your own favorite heart thumper. Or try my Bounce Back playlist.

"Some Kind of Beautiful" by Nikka Costa

"Get Up and Go" by Broadcast 3000

"We're in Your Corner" by Cornershop

"Make You Feel That Way" by Blackalicious

"32 Flavors" by Alana Davis

"Can't Feel My Face" by The Weeknd

"Everyday" by Dave Matthews Band

"Time of Our Lives" by Pitbull featuring Ne-Yo

"Emotional Rescue" by The Rolling Stones

"If He Tries Anything" by Ani DiFranco

"The Shining" by Badly Drawn Boy

WEDNESDAY

THURSDAY
Day Off!

It's your day off! Go with the flow. Allow your day to unfold to you and expand you. Remember that your body does its best repair work when you are resting or sleeping. Your muscles rebuild themselves on your day off, so this is where you get strong!

THURSDAY'S PLAYLIST: Pause

For your enjoyment, I've included an old favorite of mine for your day off. (It might just get you moving anyway.)

"Solsbury Hill" by Peter Gabriel

"Hole in the Bucket" by Spearhead

"Erotic City" by Prince and the Revolution

"Build It Up, Tear It Down" by Fatboy Slim

"Tear You Apart" by She Wants Revenge

"Remember Me" by Blue Boy

"Tennessee" by Arrested Development

"Rock and Roll Part 2" by Gary Glitter

"All Apologies" by Nirvana

"Lose Yourself" by Eminem

"Babe, We're Gonna Love Tonite" by Lime

FRIDAY

Let Go Yoga Routine: Yin Yoga Practice

40–50
MINUTES

Relax and stretch today with some Yin yoga. Yin yoga targets the fascia, tendons, and ligaments—where emotions and tension are held in the body. This routine will help to release all of that, allowing you to unwind and let go. Being in a pose for an extended period temporarily cuts off the blood flow to a part of your body; then, when you emerge from that pose, that area gets flooded with blood and nutrients.

Each pose should be held for 2–5 minutes. Since these are longer holds, there are fewer poses. In yin yoga there is no pushing—you want to find stillness. There's no need to force the pose at all. If you have any discomfort, lessen the depth of the pose. There is no right or wrong; you simply find the position that suits your body and allow yourself to relax completely. In each pose, look for ways to support yourself and your comfort so that you can relax and let go. Simply be. Allow your body to settle, and sense the nervous system as it begins to unwind.

If you would like a cardio accompaniment on this day, I recommend a 30–60 minute walk.

BUTTERFLY POSE

Come to a seated position and bring the soles of your feet together. Slide them forward to wherever feels right today. Take a few deep breaths. When you're ready, lift up and fold your body forward over your legs. You may be able to fold all the way down, or you may just lean forward with your forehead just above your feet. Find resistance and honor it by stopping when you feel it. Breathe to calm your mind. Hold this pose for 3 minutes. This pose opens the hips and the lower back.

The journey is in finding your edge.

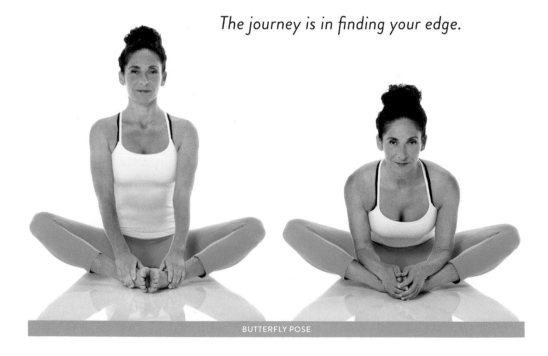

BUTTERFLY POSE

FORWARD FOLD

Extend your legs out in front of you and allow your body to fold forward. If you have a bolster or a pillow, you can place it on your thighs and allow your head or torso to be supported as you lean forward. Relax your jaw. Stay present to your breath. Hold the pose for 3 minutes. When you come out, you can wiggle your legs out in front of you to release the stretch.

There is nowhere to go.
Just being where you are right now is perfect.

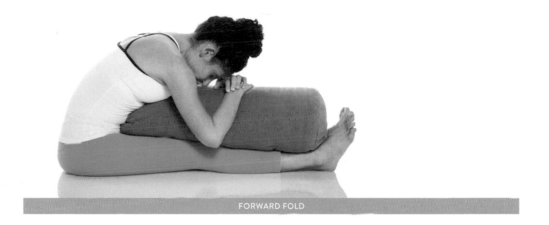

FORWARD FOLD

Counter Pose: Bring your palms behind you and raise your hips up into Reverse Table Top. Inhale and exhale, moving your body up and down 2–3 times. Loosen your legs by bending at the knees and doing a windshield wiper motion, dropping your knees from side to side.

DRAGONFLY POSE

Extend your legs open in a wide-legged split. Elevate your hips by propping yourself up with a folded blanket underneath your butt. Use blocks in front of you to rest your elbows on for support, or bring your forearms to the floor if that works for you.

Many times feelings or emotions arise from the discomfort of a pose. Hold for 3 minutes.

When you're in the position for a long period, your body may need some help getting the circulation going again. So after releasing the pose, pull the skin at the backs of your knees and rub the underside of your thighs.

Just be with what is and things will easily resolve themselves.

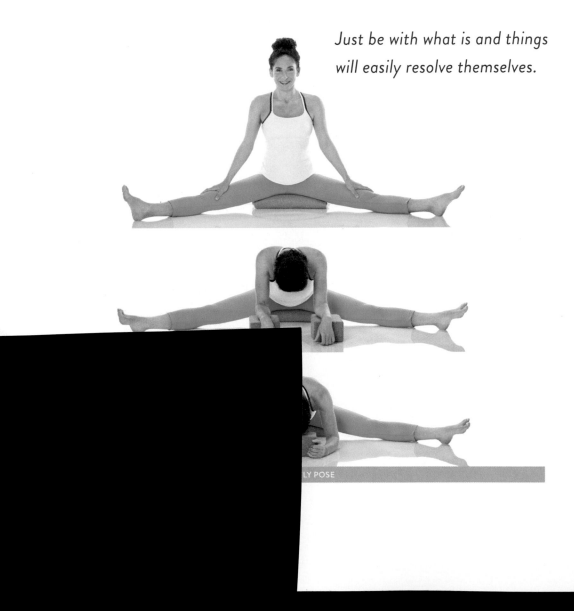

LY POSE

SPHINX POSE

Roll over onto your belly. Place your elbows underneath your shoulders. (Or, if your back is tight, you may extend the palms farther forward to get a milder backbend.) Find what works for you. Lift your chest so you're in a mini backbend. Encourage your shoulders away from your ears and then let go. After about 90 seconds, lower your torso down and rest your head to one side.

Find stillness.

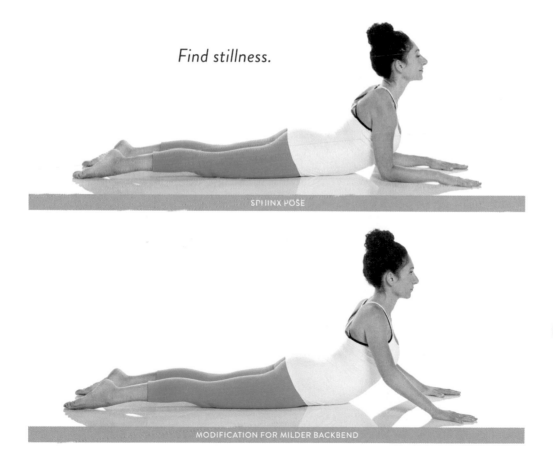

SPHINX POSE

MODIFICATION FOR MILDER BACKBEND

FRIDAY

Place one palm on top of the other and rest your head on your crossed arms. Then slide your right knee out to the side, opening up the hips and inner thighs. This is also very healthy for your kidneys. After 1 minute, release the right leg. Come up into a higher Sphinx onto your elbows.

Simply be and breathe.

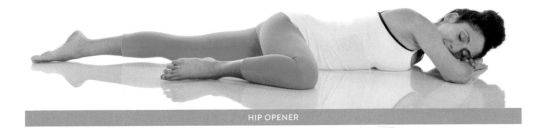

HIP OPENER

SEAL POSE

Note: Don't do this pose unless you feel comfortable. Don't push yourself.

With your hips on the floor, place your palms on the mat to lift the chest and heart. If there is pressure on your lower back, lower back down to Sphinx Pose.

Lower yourself down, rest your head to the other side, and draw your left knee up toward your underarm so you're in a hip opener. Hold this for 1 minute and then release the leg.

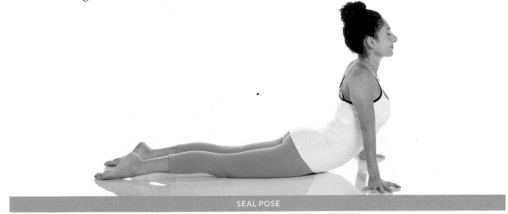

SEAL POSE

CHILD'S POSE

Shift your hips back to settle toward your heels. With toes together and knees wide apart, allow your belly and breath to soften and fill the space. Your arms can be down by the sides with palms flipped upward or outstretched in front of you with palms flat down on the mat. Your forehead and tip of the nose should lightly touch the mat. Feel your weight sinking down. Breathe deeply. Allow your jaw to go slack and bring your breath in to fill your entire back and ribs, all the way down to the kidneys. Settle here for 3 minutes.

When you are ready, rise up for a moment into Downward-Facing Dog.

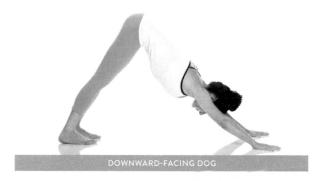

DOWNWARD-FACING DOG

Allow any tension to drain right out of you.

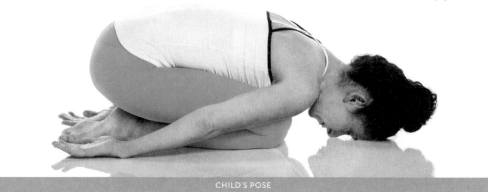

CHILD'S POSE

FRIDAY

PIGEON POSE

Step your right foot forward and bring your right knee to the ground toward your right wrist; your right heel should be on the floor toward your left hip crease. If you feel no tension in the knee, flex your foot and mindfully slide your foot forward. This is a direction for guidance, not a goal. If you have any stress on your knee joint, bring your foot closer to your hip. Slide your left leg straight back and keep your hips squared to the mat. If your right buttock is not on the floor, roll up a blanket for support and place it beneath your buttock. Fold forward and use the support of a yoga brick underneath your forehead, or come all the way down to the floor, perhaps with your palms stacked on top of each other and your head resting on your hands. Hold for 3 minutes.

Focus on relaxing and breathing

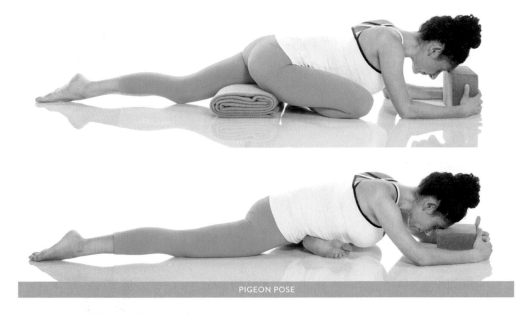

PIGEON POSE

Return to Downward-Facing Dog. Walk out the calves by stretching and bending one knee and then the other. Repeat on the other side for 3 minutes.

Extend both legs in front of you for a 30-second Forward Bend to balance out your hips.

RECLINING TWIST

Come to a supine position, draw your right knee into your chest, and extend your left leg along the floor. Extend your right arm out in line with your shoulder with the palm facing up and shift your hips slightly to the right. Place your left hand on the outside of your right knee and inhale deeply. As you exhale drop the right knee over to the left and turn your head to the right. Try to keep both shoulder blades on the mat as you breathe here. Remain here for 3 minutes and then switch sides and repeat on the other side.

Feel your stretch.

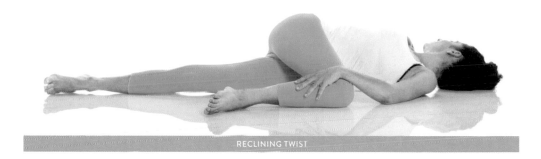

RECLINING TWIST

Counter Pose: Hug both knees into your chest.

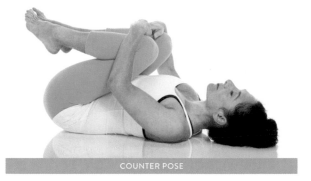

COUNTER POSE

SUPPORTED BRIDGE POSE

You will need a yoga brick for Supported Bridge Pose. Using a yoga brick will allow you to open your chest and heart. Lie on your back with your knees bent and soles of the feet on the floor, parallel to each other. Press your feet down to peel your spine off the mat and slide the block underneath your lower back so that it's supporting your sacrum, just underneath your tailbone. Play around with what position feels stable. You may use the brick at the second or third level. I like to use the block horizontally (level 2). Rest your arms out to the sides about a foot away from your hips, with your palms facing upward. Stay here for 3 minutes.

SUPPORTED SHOULDER STAND

From Supported Bridge Pose (with yoga brick), raise your legs in the air with bent knees. Once you feel stable, straighten them. Remain here for 3 minutes, allowing the blood flow to reverse from this supported position. Slowly lower down by bending the knees, then place your feet on the mat, pressing down to raise your hips up. Remove the block and then slowly, one vertebra at a time, lower down; hug your knees in and rock gently from side to side.

Focus on your breathing and how supported you feel. Just let yourself go.

SUPPORTED BRIDGE POSE

SUPPORTED SHOULDER STAND

SAVASANA/CORPSE POSE

With legs extended, and palms flipped upward, allow your feet to flop open to the sides and take a deep breath in. On the exhale, press the shoulders away from the ears and take up as much space with your breath as you can. This is your final resting pose; you can remain here anywhere from 3–10 minutes.

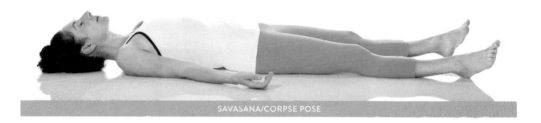

SAVASANA/CORPSE POSE

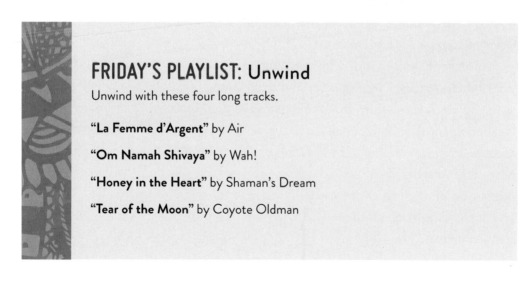

FRIDAY'S PLAYLIST: Unwind

Unwind with these four long tracks.

"La Femme d'Argent" by Air

"Om Namah Shivaya" by Wah!

"Honey in the Heart" by Shaman's Dream

"Tear of the Moon" by Coyote Oldman

FRIDAY

SATURDAY

Get Strong Yogalosophy Routine

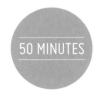

50 MINUTES

I developed Yogalosophy, my signature hybrid-yoga routine, as the answer to a call. Yoga is awesome, but my clients wanted a little something extra. So I accessed the powerful healing and strengthening benefits of yoga and paired them with complementary toners—which engage the smaller, lesser-used muscle groups—to help you get into optimal shape in the minimal amount of time. I have updated this routine and added light hand weights, so the outcome is maximum benefits with minimal effort! If you don't have weights or choose not to use them, simply follow the routine by doing 2 sets of each pair of movements.

This hybrid yoga routine with the addition of weights will stretch and tone your body, plus strengthen your muscles and build strong bones. Not only will this build your character, it will show you that, just when you think you want to give up, *that* is the moment your body is making a change. But, that said, this routine can accommodate any level of fitness, so don't worry if you're not already a yogini or have never taken a yoga class. Just take your time, breathe, do your best to get aligned properly, and be patient with yourself. It takes time to gain strength. The more you practice, the more comfortable you will be in the positions. Soon, you'll see your stamina increase.

turned in toward your body. Extend your right arm out
down like a Monkey Arm, and lower it down with contro
arm. Do 8 reps on each side.

Calf Raises + Side Lateral Raises: Hold your weights with p
As you lift your heels up for calve raises, extend both arm
at the level of your shoulders; then, as you lower your he
arms down by your sides. Repeat 8 times, then pulse the
extended at shoulder height.

8 reps + 8 pulses

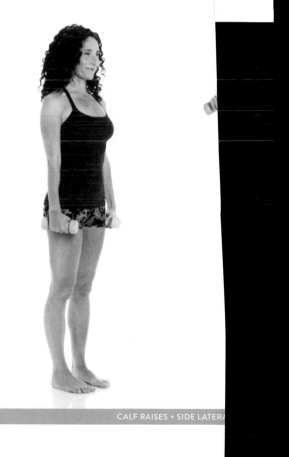

CALF RAISES + SIDE LATER/

r or hip-width apart, extend your arms by your ears, palms
your hips down into an imaginary chair. Shift your body
u look at your knees you can still see your toes. Lift your
our thighs.

der than hip-width. Lower your butt back and down to
utes and inner thighs to lift up and straighten your legs.
at your knees are aligned over your toes and that your
Do 8 reps, then pulse for 8.

8 reps + 8 pulses

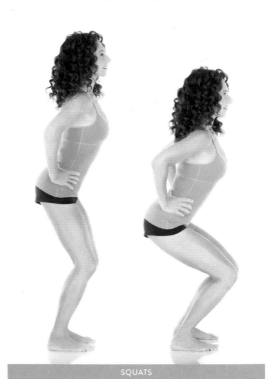

SQUATS

8 reps + 8 pulses both sides

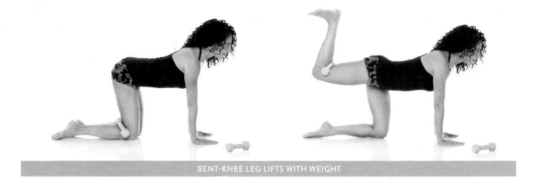

BENT-KNEE LEG LIFTS WITH WEIGHT

CAT/COW POSE/SIDE LEG LIFTS

Cat/Cow Pose: From all fours, find a neutral spine for a couple of breaths. Soften your ribs toward your spine (you can do this by exhaling sharply; feel the breath draw the ribs in) and find the natural extension from your spine out through the top of your head. On an inhale, arch your back. Rolling your shoulders back and down to engage the lateral muscles that run down the side of the body, lift your chin up; at the same time, lift the sit bones up. This is an expansion of the lungs, rib cage, and chest. On an exhale, push your palms toward the floor and tilt your tailbone under, making your torso concave. Lower your chin to your chest and lift your navel toward your spine. Inhale while arching and exhale while contracting, like a Halloween cat.

alternate 4 reps each

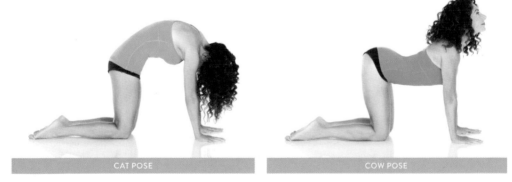

CAT POSE

COW POSE

SATURDAY

Side Leg Lifts: Place your forearms on the mat. Tuck your pelvis. Place your right hand out to the right for support. With your leg bent at a 90° angle, lift your right leg straight out to the side and then lower it to meet your left knee.

Come back to all fours and Cat/Cow 4 times. Repeat all on the left side, then return to Cat/Cow for another four reps of each.

8 reps + 8 pulses both sides

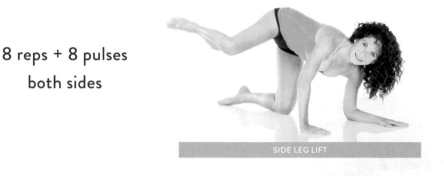

SIDE LEG LIFT

SIDE LEG LIFTS WITH WEIGHT IN CROOK OF KNEE

Side Leg Lifts with Weight in Crook of Knee: Place your hand weight securely in the crook of your bent right knee. Place your right hand on the floor out to your right side for support. Keeping your legs bent at a 90° angle, raise your right leg straight out to the side. Lower the right knee to meet the left knee.

Remove the weight and repeat Cat/Cow, then switch sides, placing the weight securely in the crook of the left knee.

8 reps + 8 pulses both sides

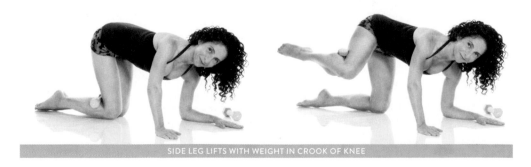

SIDE LEG LIFTS WITH WEIGHT IN CROOK OF KNEE

CONNECT (MEDITATION)

Sit in a comfortable cross-legged position with your spine straight, ideally with your hips above your knees. (MODIFICATION: Or, sit in a chair with feet planted on the floor.) Place the tops of your hands on your knees so that your palms are open.

Meditation is mindful breathing, so simply place your awareness on your breath. Notice your connection to the physical sensations and the feelings that arise.

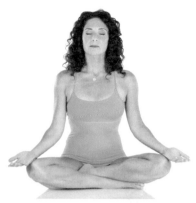

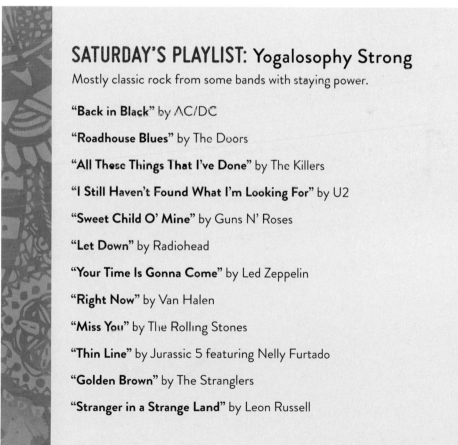

SATURDAY'S PLAYLIST: Yogalosophy Strong

Mostly classic rock from some bands with staying power.

"Back in Black" by AC/DC

"Roadhouse Blues" by The Doors

"All These Things That I've Done" by The Killers

"I Still Haven't Found What I'm Looking For" by U2

"Sweet Child O' Mine" by Guns N' Roses

"Let Down" by Radiohead

"Your Time Is Gonna Come" by Led Zeppelin

"Right Now" by Van Halen

"Miss You" by The Rolling Stones

"Thin Line" by Jurassic 5 featuring Nelly Furtado

"Golden Brown" by The Stranglers

"Stranger in a Strange Land" by Leon Russell

SATURDAY

PART TWO

The Weekly Companion to Emotional Wellness

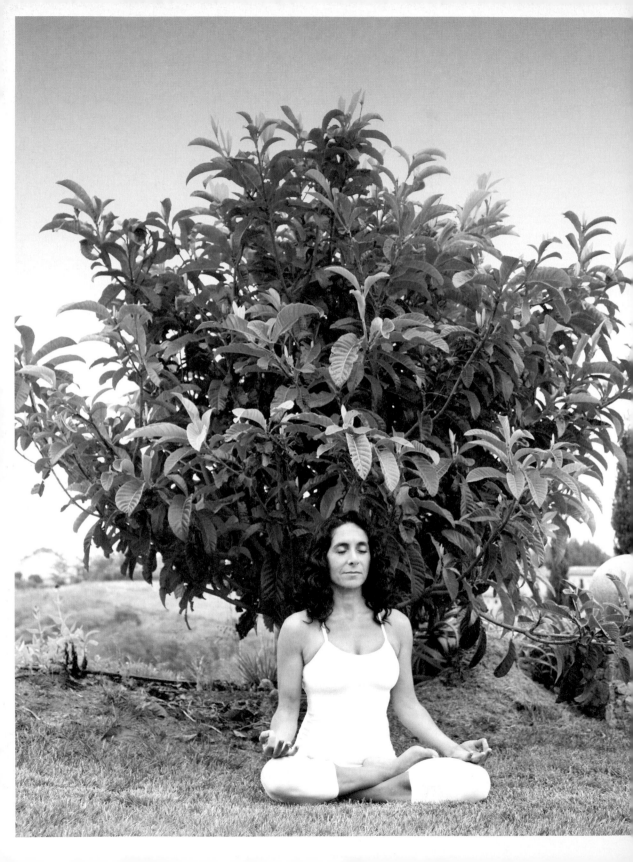

WEEK 1

Claim Your Solitude

Taking the first step toward healing your heart is not always clear. If it were, everyone would do it. But, ironically, it's not complicated. Moving toward resolution requires attention to a simple notion, and it's what we'll focus on this week: love yourself and love what is. Accept and welcome all of you, including how you feel right now.

That's right. Let everything be okay right where you are. In pain. Heartbroken. Depressed. You fill in the blank. Though you may struggle to avoid or eliminate any challenging feelings you're having, resistance is truly futile. Things don't need to be any different than they are. You don't have to be perfect. You don't have to feel great, happy, or over it. There are no wrong feelings. Everything is as it should be.

Heartbreak makes you human. It's a gift that allows you to have compassion for others who are hurting, makes you vulnerable enough to receive help from others, and reconnects you with a force that is much greater than yourself and that keeps you going even when you don't have the energy or strength to do so yourself. This universal feeling is a part of life, yet it is difficult to accept it and you avoid it because it hurts like the first time every time!

But here's the truth of it: acceptance is the basis of all growth and healing. It is the key to contentment. In *Yogalosophy: 28 Days to the Ultimate Mind-Body Makeover*, I wrote about accepting the body as already perfect, and that when I accepted my body as is, it fell into shape quite naturally and without effort. I believe the same is true of the heart, which must also be experienced as perfect in its mournful state. Rather than trying to rid yourself of the pain, focus on embracing the fullness of your heart as is, with all of its complex and human emotions. Acceptance makes no demands. It doesn't need anything to be any particular way. Its only requirement is honesty.

This week your job is to care for yourself and cherish the unique being that you are, right in this moment, and to learn to work with your own individual attributes to thrive and open your heart to the magical gift within you. The exercises in this chapter will help you learn how to get there. I should know. The path you'll follow is one I discovered by walking it myself.

It's no coincidence that as I embarked upon authoring this book I was struggling with the breakup of an eight-year relationship. The old saying goes, you teach what you need to learn, and I am learning. I was only six months into the breakup when I began this book.

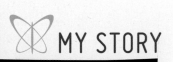 ## MY STORY

▓▓▓▓▓▓▓ nt to moving forward through the unknowable terrain on the
▓▓▓▓▓▓▓ gh there were strong signs that we were incompatible, I couldn't
▓▓▓▓▓▓▓ ove and even like between us, plus the seeming desire for the
▓▓▓▓▓▓▓ a relationship that simply wasn't right for me. I was unable to
▓▓▓▓▓▓▓ nd settle into this idea that all is as it should be, and that happy
▓▓▓▓▓▓▓ what they want, but want what they have.
▓▓▓▓▓▓▓ oting person. I want what I want! It takes me a lot of struggle
▓▓▓▓▓▓▓ lease my perception of what should be and accept what is.
▓▓▓▓▓▓▓ failure to me. But on a recent beach walk it occurred to me that when I give up it's as if I'm offering my problem "up" to the universe. It's essentially me saying, "I don't know what's best, but maybe you do, Universe. So I give it to you." Before I give up and before I settle into acceptance, I usually struggle pretty hard to avoid my feelings. I would so much rather blame something, figure it out, or think my feelings away than sink into the unsavory and all-too-human emotions of sadness, disappointment,

and especially anger that inevitably come with life's twists and turns. But my natural tendency to stave off my feelings is actually the most deadening action I could take. What I've learned this time around is that I must first become still enough to feel. So, how do I do stillness? There is no doing. There is simply sitting with the discomfort. It simply comes down to: "Don't just do something, sit there."

One of my favorite ways to avoid my feelings is to deny them by living in my imagination. Perhaps my penchant for fantasy started when I was a little girl, when I dreamed about the way things could be if my parents could get along. If only we were like other families. I could be a daddy's girl and feel protected. My parents would be like-minded and we would all be a team! In other words, if my parents were completely different people, maybe their marriage would have worked out.

As a product of divorce, I desire to fix things and make them better—back to the way they had been before. This deeply engrained belief in reconciliation echoed forward into my own relationships. I believed that "if only . . ." there had been no other woman, or if I could learn to be less irritated by messiness, or if I were more accomplished, maybe a *New York Times*–bestselling author, then somehow my relationship would work out.

Or better yet, if I wished hard enough he would change. He would come to realize that he truly did love me, and wanted to create a life with me and spend our days together. He would see that I was his best friend and that his heart was with me. The only trouble with that is that his heart was with me when we were *not* together—but each time we returned to the relationship, his heart would wander elsewhere . . . and so the merry-go-round went and went. The only way to get off: acceptance. I had to accept him exactly as he was. I also had to accept my own needs. In the cold, hard light of acceptance, these two truths were not a match.

For six months after the breakup, I resisted claiming my solitude. Solitude meant taking the time to go inward and savor being alone with and getting to know myself all over again. It meant claiming my current place in the universe. What I wanted instead was to feel better, and to be healed and fixed immediately. But then I committed to feeling all of my emotions as they arose. Sitting with the feelings. Sometimes crying, sometimes walking and crying, sometimes talking to a friend and crying. Did I mention crying? Of course there was the usual Facebook stalking, and checking up. Only my ex didn't post very often, so that was a dead end. Then there was the need to be alone where I cried and cried on the shores of my treasured Santa Monica beaches, and then the need to be around people, which would promptly disappear the moment I was around others, which left me feeling pretty awkward.

But where was my anger? When I was a teenager and studying in acting class, I will never forget my teacher saying: if you cannot access your anger, you cannot access your other emotions. This was ironic, considering my journey as an actress led me to New York

City during a life-altering moment when I was fifteen years old. When I left on my exciting new journey to star in a prestigious Broadway show by Neil Simon, I had no idea that I was leaving behind the first chapter of my life. While I was embarking on an exciting career, my entire family fell apart from my father's affair and my parents' separation, the school that I cherished closed, and life as I knew it had all but dissolved. I cannot even recall the last day that I lived in the same home with my own father. Somewhere, underneath all of this loss, there was a feeling I could not pinpoint but that has motivated me nonetheless.

That feeling is anger. Anger has never been easy for me. I battle with my anger, and even as a child my anger would become shrouded behind a veil of tears. As an adult, rage replaced anger. Its expression was more of a buildup, but not a free flow. It must be some-where inside, but where?

Eventually, I learned how to watch my anger. I am now way more attentive to my pro-cess when I sit as a witness knowing that I am the science experiment.

One of the great takeaways I've garnered from yoga is the ability to cultivate the "wit-ness," which is the ability to observe life's twists and turns without judgment. This time my sorrow has a container and a purpose. This time, as I observed myself, I decided I was going to share with you the gems I found along the way. I was committed. Once I knew that I was not alone, not completely alone—because I had this awesome observer within me, and the "me" that was going to go through this and share with you in real time—I could surrender to what would be the best breakup process of my life.

We will go into this more later, but for now let's just say I am not good at breakups. I generally get more deeply attached to the other person than most humans I've met do. I am learning to accept that in myself.

I am also in acceptance that I have very large feelings and emotions. I am the type of person who tends to suppress my true feelings and intuition, so I am practicing acceptance and expression of my feelings. At one time I thought this expression may appear to be an "overreaction." But if I take responsibility and own my truth, it's not. Instead, it's my pathway to honoring and taking care of my feelings on my own, to feeling all of my feelings without laying them on anyone else's doorstep. With acceptance comes stillness, even in the midst of all of the emotion.

This stillness provided me more than peaceful moments while in the eye of my emo-tional storm. It gave me the mental clarity to see my truth—and tend to it. My "truth" came to me in the most unexpected way this time. It was a revelation, and it came after a complete standstill. Here's what happened.

As I was seeking to release and let go of this on- and on-again relationship, I knew that I needed more space. I was craving space. So I walked on the beach. I received incredibly slow and intimate bodywork. I identified that what I was looking for in a person was that they had all the time in the world for me. So that is what I sought from myself. I cleared my plate of my private clients, finding other teachers for them. I detached from most friend-ships and disentangled myself from everyone else's projects and requests. I received great support from cranialsacral/polarity therapy, which primarily recalibrated my energy, but also opened me further to talking it out. I got support when I needed it. What I discovered I really wanted was a death ritual: something that would redefine letting go in a way that would allow me to experience it.

This was all leading up to the winter holidays, and although I planned to get away, I felt so utterly stagnant. I was feeling depressed and dull, lethargic, and lacking excitement toward anything.

Then one night, when I was having a particularly difficult time sleeping, something dawned on me. My digestive system had been sluggish and had come to a complete stand-still. For over a month. Nothing. It's not like I didn't know this was going on, but since being "regular" had never been an issue before, I figured that my body would take care of itself. Then, as if a veil had been lifted, I remembered a story my friend Tricia had shared with me several months before when I asked about her ongoing back pain. It turned out it was her colon. She had dehydrated her system and had become totally backed up. All at once I realized that this was what was happening to me! I had been slowly dehydrating myself over time. Drinking coffee and very little water, going to the sauna daily, sweating in hot yoga and Spinning . . . and not caring to eat hydrating foods. No wonder I had not been hungry or even interested in any new experiences—there was no room! This aha moment came to me on Christmas Eve. Needless to say, there was nobody available to help me on that day. I had finally come to a standstill where I was face-to-face with myself. There were no distractions to hide the reality of what my state of being was in that present moment. My mentality snapped and I completely switched gears. Prior to experiencing the awakening, I had been self-neglecting to the point of becoming very ill. I began to take immediate ac-tion with colon hydrotherapy and literally babying myself by sipping a gallon of water daily and consuming only soups, smoothies, and mush that resembled, well, baby food. I had been looking for a death ritual and I had found one: I was dying inside. Nothing physical or mental was moving until I had the epiphany. Had I not seen an old friend and had she not shared transparently with me, had I not cleared the decks of work and social commitments, I may not have had the realization. Once this came to me, everything else quickly came into a very clear focus.

Certain experts say that all of the emotions are processed in the colon. We digest our experiences through our bodies, and so my colon was communicating with me. My only job at the moment was to take care of and baby myself, and to share my self-love healing experience with you in this book. As I observed the seriousness of my condition, all of my past self-inflicted childhood eating disorder issues came forth and I realized that, on some subconscious level, I had been dehydrating myself on purpose. It was the same part that starved myself as a young girl. Suddenly the veil was lifted, and the angry part of myself that was withholding, neglectful, and even punishing was revealed. Of course I had chosen to be with a partner who didn't have time for me, who wouldn't fully embrace our union, and who delayed commitment for another time in the future. That was what I had been doing to myself all along. In an instant, I understood that my former relationship was a reflection of self-neglect that arose from a deep-seated anger, and I was now humbled and ready for true change. My anger uses the silent treatment, and it positions for power by not participating. My anger looks more like a cement wall than a scary monster. I started to dialogue a little with it, and realized that my fear is so connected with my anger and that it's simply a hidden, creative part of myself that wants to be recognized and seen. As with most of our shadow qualities, when we invite them into the room and shed a little light, they are not so ugly after all.

Everyone's experience in dealing with distress is personal, physically and emotionally. You surely have your own story to tell. But I can guarantee you that your story will be different, more illustrious, and evolved by the end of the next twelve weeks.

Here you are, at the beginning of this book, looking for answers or help in moving past a difficult time in your life. What do you do, right here, right now? Only this: tuck aside your desire to fix everything, to feel better, to move on. Instead, claim this moment of solitude. Consider it your opportunity to become a certified "self-love" expert. That's right, certified.

You are the only one who can certify you as a self-love expert. Nobody outside you can know if you are truly doing self-love to the level of expertise that is required. You will know when it is true. And you will find the pathway to that truth through acceptance of where you are at this moment.

This week, love yourself and love what is. You don't have to be perfect. Things don't need to be any different than they are. You were born with a certain genetic makeup, certain emotional, mental, and physical needs, and you have a purpose that is uniquely yours. Your job is to care for yourself and cherish the unique being that you are, to learn to work with your particular brand of awesome and thrive. The Self-Love Checklist will help you to open your heart to the magical truth that you are enough as you are.

LOVE MOVEMENT: SPINNING

Cardio activity channels emotional energy into physical action. This can be especially effective for releasing anger. Spinning was an excellent jump-start for me when I was thawing out from my childhood pain. When I got on my first Spinning bike in 1991, the suppressed anger finally had a physical outlet. In the early 1990s, after years of fitness classes, high-impact aerobics, a variety of yoga styles, ton-

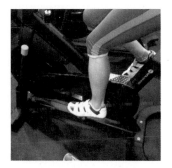

ing classes, step classes, dance, hip-hop, and more, I found, to my amazement, that Spinning accessed the key to my self-awareness and to the healing of my eating disorder. Spinning gave me a way in to my center and my desire to move, while connecting me to a deep stillness at my core. It informed my yoga practice and allowed me to cultivate "the witness."

The year 1991 was pivotal for me, as my wounds were reopened. I was extremely vulnerable from the impact of two unlikely incidents that cut me right open. In 1989, a dear friend I had met while working on a television series "My Sister Sam," actress Rebecca Schaeffer, was shot and killed by a stalker only two weeks after our last visit. Her murder was widely televised and I became numb with disbelief at this tragic loss. My heart ached and my mind kept returning to our last meeting. It was this incident that caused me to reassess opening myself up to being public the way I had been doing through acting. This was followed by a personal incident just a year later in 1990 where I was physically beaten and almost raped and my roommate was raped. Needless to say, I had experienced a lot that could have brought me way down without return. But there is a depth of intimacy with the self and a survival instinct that I became inextricably in touch with. It was in this place that I found my edge and my resilience. In many ways, these incidents gave me an inner strength I did not know I had. Channeling this energy into actual movement on the Spinning bike connected me with a power that has fueled my life and given it meaning.

Spinning provides a place—in the middle of the intensity of great emotions—to channel all that energy while sitting still in the moment. Since the exercise is so simple (having only three hand positions and five movements), it doesn't require a lot of technical attention, so it allows a true investigation into the thoughts, feelings, and emotions that come into play in the moments of strain, stress, and intensity. It's amazing to feel the power of that stabilizing still point amidst great action. In other words: "Don't just do something, sit there!" The beauty of emotions is that they are fuel and energy. Emotions put our energy into motion. It doesn't matter if you are angry or deeply sad, as either emotion will ignite your legs and you will transcend the feeling itself. For years I have witnessed many people with broken hearts find their way in my spin class. The catharsis that comes is unparalleled, and I will speak for myself when I say that I have gotten very intimate with a difficult process by showing up to the bike and motivating daily. To see where my edge is and where I go when I think I can't take it. I became the observer on the bike and that translated to my yoga. So be fearless and try a Spinning class this week. But as always, you know best. If Spinning is not your thing, try any active class. Remain connected to your center.

ERIKA'S STORY

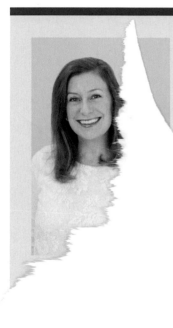

I met my friend Erika Lenkert in 2007, when we were both spokespeople for a women's empowerment initiative for a sports beverage. I was the "Inspire" expert and Erika was the "Connection" expert. Something like the real girl's Martha Stewart, Erika was known for her ability to create connection instantly—and that she did. It was ⁻tant love for me. As an empowered woman herself,
         has strengthened me with plenty of encourage-
             support. When I didn't know I could write a
               me I could. When we had conversations,
                  ᵗʰ me about her own life. Ever
                      ᵃʳner as much wisdom
                         ᵉ contribution

Erika

At forty-seven years old, I thought I knew heartbreak. I'd experienced the deaths of beloved people and pets, gone through divorce, and rode out the searing, festering emotions surrounding betrayal by close friends and family. I was pretty sure I could find my way to the other side of anything. Until him. He came out of nowhere, and just like that, I couldn't imagine life without him, my true soul mate. And I didn't have to. He handed me the moon and the promise of happily ever after.

Perhaps it was the glow of love-drunk moonlight that shrouded the warning signs, even though they were giant, neon, and perpetually flashing, but I never saw it coming until it was upon me: a pain so piercing, so all-consuming that everything else fell away and I was little more than a shell of myself, no longer living in the moment but trapped in my mind, lost in grief, and repeatedly replaying the scenario. That was me for a full year. No longer a sunshine spirit, no longer of the moment. I lived in the past, a modern version of Dickens's Miss Havisham.

I can't tell you what snapped me out of it. I did everything to get there—yoga, meditation, beating pillows, running, therapy, healthy eating, sleeping, dating, hanging with friends, performing rituals where I imagined sawing through the thick roots attaching my aching heart to his. Though there was some movement, nothing truly worked.

Then one day, I woke up and the weight was gone. Just like that. The perpetual, grueling conversation in my head quieted. I found myself laughing—a lot and freely. I once again became energized by the force of everyday beauty, like the rustle of the wind in the trees or the sun streaming through the morning clouds.

I'm not sure I'll ever be entirely over it. But I am beginning to see the gifts the experience gave me, and they are rich. Rumi was right: "You have to keep breaking your heart until it stays open." This doozy of a heartbreak cracked mine into a million pieces. Now those fragments are everywhere, coating my perspective with tenderness, compassion, and gratitude in a way I could never have experienced otherwise.

Open, accepting, forgiving, and more fragile and resilient than I've ever been, I believe I am left with the truest love of all.

HEART-HEALING MEDITATION: SIMPLE, MINDFUL BREATHING

A great description I've heard about meditation goes something like this: "Inhale. Exhale. Continue." You may have heard a lot about mindfulness recently, for it has become a catchphrase these days. What is mindfulness? Simply put, mindfulness asks you to come to the present moment. This is easier said than done, especially when you're in the process of letting go of old habits and patterns represented by your recent loss. Left to its own devices, the mind wanders. The point of mindfulness is to direct your awareness away from the thoughts or the "monkey mind" and back to the experience where you can anchor yourself in the now. Of course your mind will wander; the idea is to watch when that happens and to make that conscious. Just like any muscle, the more you practice, the stronger it will be. Simply allow whatever comes up to come up. Do not judge it as good or bad. Returning to the observation and just noticing, cultivating the witness, is something that I promise will become your best friend.

To practice simple, mindful breathing, find a comfortable seated position. Set your timer for twenty minutes.

As you sit in silence, begin to focus on your breath moving in and out of your nose. Become aware of the pause and the space in between the breaths. After the inhalation and then after the exhalation. This pause is where all the action is. Notice the sounds in the room, the neighbor outside having a phone conversation, the *whiz* of a passing car, birds chirping. Whatever is there, notice. Notice the sensation of your skin. Is there a light breeze? Are your palms slightly clammy? Bring your mind back to your breath. Notice the thoughts as they arise. Just like clouds going by, simply see that thought as a cloud. Let it pass. Pass no judgment; there is no good or bad. Observe the present moment. This is cultivating the witness and harnessing your mind back into this moment.

LOVE NOTES: AFFIRMATION

Create your own prayer or affirmation that allows you to ask for help or reset yourself. Or use this one: "I completely love and accept myself."

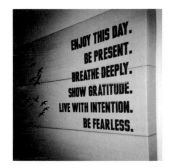

My affirmation has become "Claim your solitude." At first I did not want to be by myself, and I wanted to immediately replace the old relationship with something else. But once I surrendered, something shifted within me. Now I am making all sorts of discoveries about my relationship to myself, realizing that I am quite enjoying this process and taking my space. Today, I choose to be alone and Claim My Solitude. If you feel inspired, take a few minutes to journal about your own affirmation.

RITUAL: THE "NO!" EXERCISE

In order to find your "Yes!" you must find your "No!" Many of us have been raised to be nice and try to accommodate others. This lack of boundaries can compromise your sense of self and what you truly need to thrive. When the "NO!" in you is unexpressed, it lays dormant and creates internal resistance. Here's how it goes: Stand with feet hip-width apart and knees slightly bent. Start with arms extended out in front of your body and make fists with your hands. Thrust your hips forward while pulling your bent elbows back and shouting "No!" as loudly as you can. Repeat this thrusting movement and action while shouting the word "No!" over and over again without pause for three minutes. When the time is up, stand still and feel all of the energy coursing through your body. It is very powerful to feel your anger when channeled in a positive and responsible way. Savor this feeling because anger is one of the great motivators to fuel you to move along on your journey.

The heart chakra (*anahata*), the fourth chakra, is located in the heart region of your chest. It is associated with trust, forgiveness, compassion, patience, wisdom, and emotional empowerment. This chakra bridges the spirit world and the physical world. It is through the heart that you are able to enjoy the human experience of heaven on Earth. Feeling and unconditional love are the gateway from the material world to the metaphysical world. The word *anahata* means "flawless" or "unstuck" in Sanskrit. That means your heart is flawless, and that you are perfect exactly as is. It is represented by the twelve-petal lotus flower. The heart chakra gives you a feeling of vitality for being alive and allows you to feel compassion for others and to be truly connected and interested in their well-being. Physiologically, this chakra is associated with the thoracic cavity and governs the physical heart, rib cage, blood, lungs, diaphragm, thymus gland, breasts, and esophagus. When imbalanced, it can manifest as upper back and shoulder issues, asthma, lung or heart disease, and shallow/rapid breathing. When the heart chakra is weakened you experience feelings of loneliness, hopelessness, lack of self-esteem, paranoia, jealousy, indecisiveness, fear of letting go, anxiety, mistrust, and physical heart problems. When this chakra is overactive, you may experience dependency or breathing problems, have control issues, make reckless decisions, or be overly trusting or overpromising.

A balanced and open heart chakra will read as calm, confident, and trusting of the self. One way to strengthen your heart chakra is to open yourself to the world. I'm going to help you with exercises that explore this throughout our twelve-week journey in this book. On the next page is a list of tools that we will revisit and expand upon as we move through the weeks ahead. This can bring much joy and peace to your being.

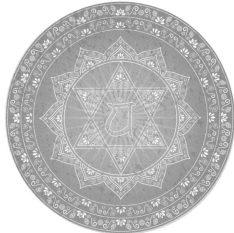

AFFIRMATIONS: "I completely love and accept myself"; "Love is everywhere"

ASK YOURSELF: "Do I love and accept myself?"

SENSE: Touch

SYSTEMS: Respiratory, circulatory, immune

FOOD: Vegetables (especially dark leafy greens!)

INNER STATE: Compassion

EMOTIONS: Trust, love

COLOR: Green (calming color: pink)

YOGA POSES: Camel, Fish, Cobra

HERBS: Thyme, Melissa

OILS/SPICES: Rose, jasmine, saffron, tarragon

FLOWER REMEDY: Chicory, red chestnut

AROMATHERAPY: Rose

METAL: Copper

GEMSTONES: Rose quartz, jade, emerald

ELEMENT: Air

NATURE: Forests and fields

CELESTIAL BODY: Venus

MOON PHASES: New and full

HEART FACT A recent study in India showed that the benefits of yoga and meditation, even after just fifteen days, yielded a lower resting pulse and lowered blood sugar, which helps to prevent heart disease.

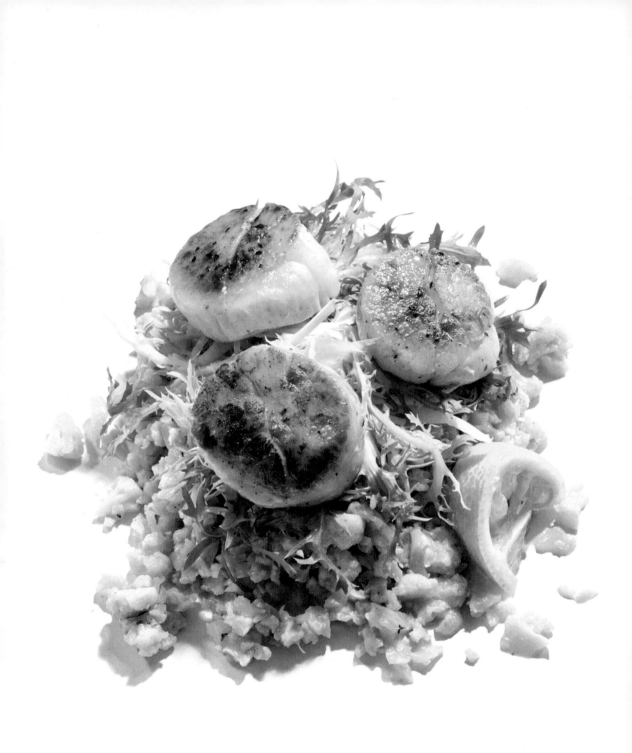

CAULIFLOWER RISOTTO WITH SAUTÉED SCALLOPS AND FRISÉE

Serves 2

Get all the rich, creamy goodness of risotto without the heavy carb guilt with this deceptively light and elegant dish. Lightning fast to make and a dream to eat, its quick-cooking cauliflower "rice"—laden with savory Parmesan and chicken stock—and delicate scallops play perfectly with the lightly citrusy tuft of frisée.

2 TEASPOONS OLIVE OIL

½ CUP CHOPPED ONION

1 CUP GLUTEN-FREE CHICKEN STOCK

1 HEAD CAULIFLOWER, FINELY CHOPPED

½ CUP GRATED PARMESAN CHEESE

6 LARGE SCALLOPS, EACH ABOUT 1½ INCHES THICK

KOSHER SALT AND FRESHLY GROUND PEPPER

2 CUPS LOOSELY PACKED FRISÉE LETTUCE

1 LEMON, QUARTERED

In a large sauté pan, heat 1 teaspoon of olive oil over medium heat. Add the onion and cook, stirring frequently to avoid browning, about 5 minutes. Add the chicken stock and continue cooking to soften the onion and reduce the liquid, about 10 minutes. Add the cauliflower and cook until tender, stirring occasionally, about 10 minutes. Stir in the Parmesan. Set aside.

Season the scallops with salt and pepper. In a small sauté pan, heat 1 teaspoon of oil over medium heat and sauté the scallops until just cooked through, about 2 minutes per side.

To serve, divide the risotto between two dinner plates, top with half the frisée, squeeze a quarter lemon over each, top with three scallops, and serve with a lemon wedge.

Recipe by Erika Lenkert; reprinted with permission from her gluten-free gourmet food publication, GFF. (Learn more at www.gffmag.com.)

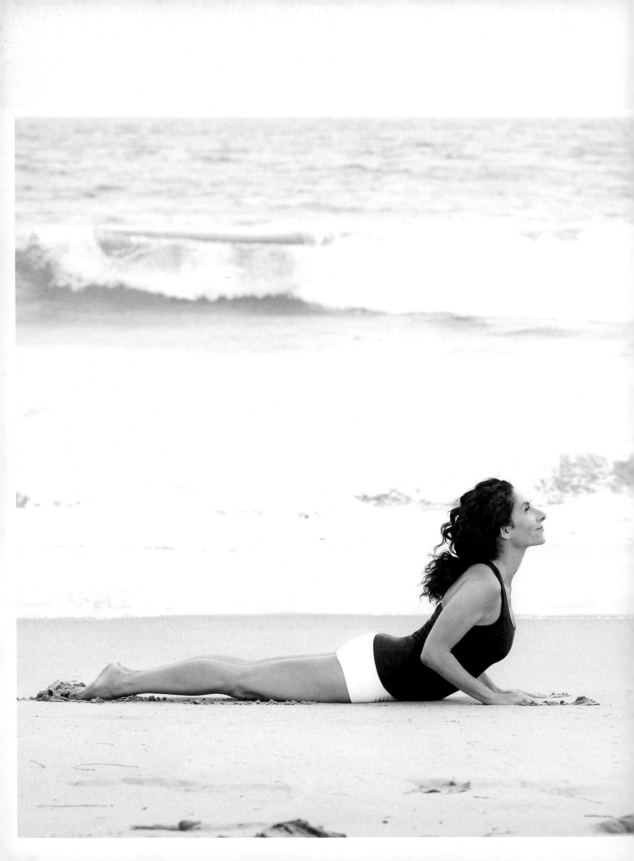

WEEK 2

Grow Down

L et me tell you something that should bring you some relief as you ponder how you're going to move through, and up, from where you are now: growing is an action that happens on its own, no matter what. And, growing does not always look like what you think it should. Take a tree as an example. A tree's branches grow, reaching toward the sunlight, stretching, and lifting upward as much as they possibly can. I call this "growing up" and liken it to the kind of directions you may think you need to move on from where you are now. Get above it. Reach upward. Move on. But what you don't see in that tree is what the roots are do-  ing. They are growing down deep into the foundation. These strong, unsung anchors are what allow the tree its reach—by giving it the stability and the grounding that is needed for it to climb to heights never reached before.

As long as a plant has proper conditions of water and sunlight, it will grow, but even sometimes when the conditions are not good there can be growth. A grapevine is a great example of this. Deprive it of water and it will produce less fruit—but the roots will grow deeper into the Earth in search of water, and the fruit will become more concentrated in flavor. These are examples of hope, and of where you are. Standing tall and deepening your connection to your roots is key to understanding that your experiences are grounding you, that you are growing around (and through) them, and that they are making you who you are—deeper, richer, more concentrated in flavor. Nature provides!

I'm not the only one who knows this is true. The results of studies conducted by A. Clinton Ober and Dr. Russell Whitten show that connecting with the Earth by walking barefoot or lying directly on the ground reduces inflammation and has health benefits related specifically to the heart and the nervous system. "Earthing" is the practice of connecting the body with the Earth by touching skin to a conductive material like wet grass, wet sand, or a river, lake, or sea. Sensing that connectivity with nature not only gives you a powerful physical charge, it also allows you to know in your soul that growth is inevitable—just by taking a simple action like walking on a sandy beach with your bare feet. There is always hope when you grow where you are planted.

So this week we'll focus on, and ritualize, growing down. We'll explore the supportive force that is a constant for each of us through grounding actions. We will plant our feet and bodies firmly on the ground, engage with nature, and explore our familial roots or history. I'll show you that, when you feel lost and adrift or falling, you can notice and appreciate that nature is right there to hold you and catch you, and that in the experience you will get more in touch with your growing foundation—and perhaps even find appreciation for the painful catalyst that brought you to this moment. ███████ don't yet understand, but there is a natural force that can ███████ state. At any moment, you can choose to rely upon this ███████ in the consistency of the Earth's cycles throughout time.

�֍ MY STORY

I thought I had it all figured out. I had watched my parents go through the breakdown of their marriage. In a way, my entire childhood was spent observing the slow deterioration of their relationship, and I studied them like the most committed student. I even took notes, in my child hand, suggesting what they might improve and how they could make more space for each other's perspective. I also thought a lot about how I could stay ahead of the game. I was determined to do it better.

As a young girl, I dreamed of having a perfect relationship when I grew up. My partner was going to value and cherish me. He would swoop in and win me over. I conjured the perfect mate, but it was a fairy tale I made up. A fantasy. Like all fairy tales, my standards were higher than mere mortals could reach—but that's what I wanted. I was determined to skip over the messy stuff. As I grew older, the way I dealt with the gulf between the reality and the ideal was to avoid serious relationships completely. Why try to relate with an actual human being when my dream was so much richer? Although I did meet one or two interesting men along the way, I thought I was better off being free than settling on a less than idyllic relationship. So much time passed that I became more invested in the control I had flying solo than in testing the romantic waters. By the time I was thirty, I had successfully accomplished my goal: I had not repeated the failed marriage of my parents. Although secretly I still longed for the love I saw in my Disney books, I didn't really believe it could happen. I was an independent woman, fully self-supporting and self-sufficient. I remained untethered by unfulfilling relationships like the ones I saw my friends having. I felt really smart. And then one day I was caught off guard. I lost my glass slipper and I fell in love.

We started as friends. He was an instructor who taught a class immediately after mine. I remember a student saying to me that he was her type, and my noting that he was definitely not my type. He kind of annoyed me—but he also made me laugh, and I made him laugh, too. He was leaving a marriage, so he was definitely off-limits and not available. I was safe to be myself! There was no immediate sign of romantic attraction. But one random day, without warning, Cupid's arrow got me. I was tricked! I fell under a deep spell, just like they write about in the fairy tales. My dream was coming true.

We were a couple for five years—his longest relationship and my first—and very early in our relationship we moved in together because it seemed logical. The universe appeared to be bringing us together in the most unlikely way. You see, he had nowhere to live and was couch surfing, for he had left his wife, and I had nowhere to live because my apartment had burned down. (Don't ask. That's a different book.) So we migrated from place to place for ten months, ultimately deciding that if we could cohabitate as gypsies and be happy, then living together in a more stable setting would be a piece of cake. It was. We lived in a tiny Santa Monica apartment and had a very sweet life together. As time went on, our romance continued to rage. It appeared as if this guy was permanently attached to my hip. He loved me completely and totally, in spite of my flaws—twenty pounds heavier, with a burned-down apartment, a broken-down car, and a singed pink tutu. It was okay with him. All of it.

I was not easy to please (I never have been). I once asked him, "Do you still love me even though I'm a mess?" and he said, "I love you *because* you're a mess." He loved me as is.

He would do anything to please me. A friend of mine made a joke that if I asked him to remove the apartment building across the street so that I could see the view, he would.

He would stop at nothing; his affections were demonstrated daily with gifts, cards, flowers, romance, and I responded with a level of affection and trust I didn't know I had.

Then in our fifth year, without warning, my perfect guy went from red hot to ice cold. He began to question his life choices and our relationship and then to withdraw into confusion. I was devastated. I felt duped by the universe. I was angry at that force for tricking me this way. And in my mind the bitter conclusion rose up: *You see, this is why I avoided relationships all my life. This is why I never wanted to fall in love.* The spell was broken.

After he left, I was overcome with physical waves of withdrawal, as if something inside me, at my core, was dead. There was a sinking, heavy feeling in my body. It was not long before I found it difficult to take a physical step forward, and soon had an injury that mirrored the way I felt inside: I threw my back out and was unable to stand up or even roll over. Talk about growing down and getting close to the ground! I felt *flattened*. I couldn't understand how this had happened to me.

It would have been easier if he'd done something to hurt me and I could have been mad at him. I might have been less adrift had he left me for another woman, or if he was a jerk during the breakup, or if he'd led me on or been mean. At least then I could have had an excuse for being angry. But that's not what happened, and so I just felt despondent—left pining and weakened. In the end, he left me for himself. It was as simple as that. He left because the relationship had simply run its course. We were no longer growing together, but I could not see that at the time.

But there is more to the story. The moment he broke up with me (over the phone), I did something completely unexpected. I dropped to my knees in a puddle of tears and started saying "thank you." I didn't know why. It was completely and utterly counterintuitive, and the opposite of what I was feeling. Yet there was a grain of truth alive in me—mysterious, but there. Perhaps it was because I had seen the ultimate outcome of my parents' divorce. Both ended up happier, with more appropriate partners, and maybe that would happen to me, too. I was saying "thank you" because on some level I knew that the breakup was *for* me. Perhaps the entire relationship had happened just so I could have this moment. But that understanding came later.

So there I was, injured and battered by external pressures. My love had flown, I'd lost my job, and my father was dying of cancer. It was a dark time. But it was also a catalyst. In an effort to go back to my roots and channel my energies properly, I decided to turn to yoga teacher's training. I knew I could not find my way by relying on others or on external circumstances. I had to go inward. I needed to stop looking outside myself for love and root into what was real and at my very core. *I needed to grow up by growing down.*

As I mentioned at the beginning of this chapter, growing down manifests in the physical and the emotional. In the physical body, growing down means literally looking down and feeling where your feet are, taking off your shoes, and walking barefoot on the sandy beach or a grassy path. It means being in contact with nature and feeling what is around you. A breeze, a spray of ocean water, even a human walking by and smiling reconnects you to the Earth. Sitting directly on the Earth or hugging a tree are other ways to connect with nature's healing field. Watching a sunrise or sunset brings you into the present moment.

Growing down also means feeling the fear that lives in your bones and blood through the DNA of your blood relatives. In my case, it's feeling the fear of family who lost their relatives in the war, the fear of getting "found out" or of perhaps there being something wrong with me simply because I was born a certain religion. My mother was born in Germany in an internment camp where her family resided after losing their relatives. My grandfather lost three brothers, a sister, and his mother in the Holocaust. Both of my grandparents were just teenagers when the war broke out, and were on the run, fighting for their lives. So in growing down I felt the fear of their loss, yet the gratitude of their survival. On my paternal side, I felt the conditioning of my father, who'd never had his own father's approval and so felt a lack of worthiness as a result. Both of these historical experiences are in my bones, and the breakup was a wonderful representation for healing the deep sense of fear and misunderstanding I held inside me. I was gifted with this relationship and its demise because it helped me to heal old genetic wounds.

Growing down empowers me to embrace and own my strengths. Growing down empowers me to being present, to understanding that I have a sound mind and many gifts that have developed and grown *because of* my weaknesses. The grace that was passed through my parents who did the best they could with what they had. Being blessed with tenacity and the gifts of circumstance.

As you enter into this week's practices, the aim is to love your foundation. What you have within you is a gift. I had no choice but to go deep into myself and find the gratitude for the present moment. Gratitude is a contrary action, and it's what saved me. It can save you, too. That surrendered "thank you," when you feel the most wounded, is the beginning of your healing. It recognizes a force that wants the best for you. It's bigger than you. It's the force of nature itself. Mother Earth actually has a heart, vibrating at a frequency that resonates with your own heart center. You are where you're supposed to be. Your foundational history brings you a special gift—as well as historical issues that are to be released back into the Earth. With gratitude, there is hope. I know that you can access that hope, too, as you grow down into your personal place on this Earth.

SELF-LOVE CHECKLIST

YOGALOSOPHY FOR INNER STRENGTH program

- ❑ **Sunday:** Be Happy Yoga
- ❑ **Monday:** Back–to–Basics Yoga
- ❑ **Tuesday:** Cardio
- ❑ **Wednesday:** Bounce Back! Yoga
- ❑ **Thursday:** Day Off
- ❑ **Friday:** Let Go Yoga
- ❑ **Saturday:** Get Strong Yogalosophy
- ❑ **Heart-Opening Pose:** Cobra
- ❑ **Love Movement:** Grounding Hike or Beach Walk
- ❑ **Heart-Healing Meditation:** Grounding Cord Meditation
- ❑ **Love Notes:** The Gratitude List
- ❑ **Ritual:** A Gift of Love
- ❑ **Strength for the Soul:** Flowers That Heal

MANTRA

I am so grateful that I am fully supported. I trust that the universe provides me with all I need.

TRACK OF THE WEEK

"Thank You" by Dido or "Thanks for the Information" by Van Morrison

HEART-OPENING POSE: COBRA

All backbends are heart openers. Anything that opens up the chest and shoulders falls into this category. I have chosen the Cobra Pose for this week because it allows you to get grounded by laying your body down low to the ground. Incorporate Cobra into your routine each day this week and shed your skin.

- Lie down on your belly and place your hands beneath your shoulders with your palms down.
- Place the tops of your feet flat on the mat.

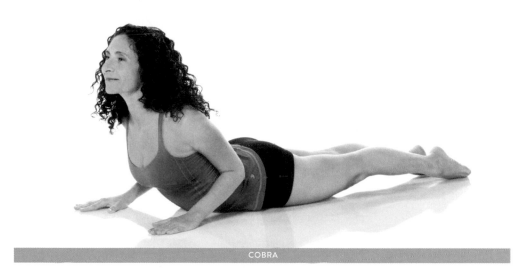

COBRA

- Tuck your tailbone and draw your belly in to protect your lower back.

- Spread your fingers equal distance. Roll your shoulders back and down. Hug your elbows in toward your rib cage.

- Open your chest, and lift your upper body off the mat while keeping your hips, legs, and feet planted to the floor. Press the tops of all ten toes into the mat.

- Hold for 5 long, slow breaths. This pose increases strength of back, arms, and shoulders, improves flexibility of the spine, and elevates your mood.

LOVE MOVEMENT: GROUNDING HIKE OR BEACH WALK

Walking on the ground is literally grounding! Hiking is both grounding and a natural activity. Choose a natural setting—a park, woods, beach, or quiet path—where you can be away from the ordinary noise and business. Leave your cell phone behind. Watch your body recalibrate itself when you choose silence and solitude. While on your hike, pay attention to nature and notice the sounds, smells, and sensations all around you. Experience a connection to your own strength and endurance. Hike for 45–90 minutes, at a pace that feels comfortable. Take your time and return to your breathing as much as you can. The present moment is your gift. Be aware. Imagine that nature is speaking to you on your

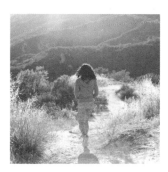

hike. Consider the positive messages you are absorbing through your surroundings. Feel your tension releasing as you let go of your fears and sorrows and allow yourself to be taken care of by your real mother: nature.

EXTRA CREDIT: WALK BAREFOOT.

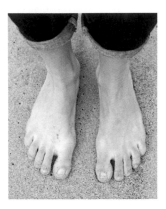

As I mentioned at the beginning of this chapter, there are recent studies showing that there are benefits from walking barefoot, such as reducing inflammation, increasing energy, reducing stress, improving blood flow, relieving tension headaches, supporting adrenal health, enabling deeper sleep, and shortening recovery time from injuries. Magical!

ALEXIS'S STORY

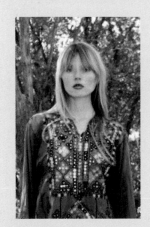

My friend Alexis Smart is a flower-remedy practitioner and homeopath living in Los Angeles. Her passion for flower remedies began after Bach flower remedies cured her of anxiety attacks after only three weeks of use. She now has her own line of Bach formulas. You can find out more about her at www.AlexisSmart.com or get her custom blends at Urban Outfitters and Free People. Alexis has been featured in magazines such as *Vogue, Elle, Vanity Fair, C, Daily Candy,* and *Lucky.* You can find Alexis's DIY flower essence remedy in the Heart Connection section on page 184.

• • •

Alexis

I met my first love, Charlie, when I was sixteen and he was twenty. He had dropped out of Dartmouth College and moved to Los Angeles, where I lived, to pursue music. He was gentle and kind, and had all the qualities I have yet to find in another man: loyalty, honesty, passion, and innocence.

But after two years together, something changed for me. I was still a kid, but he was a man, and I wasn't ready for a lifelong love. I began to feel smothered, and I broke up with him. When we parted, he said that he would always love me, and that if I ever changed my mind, even if it was in twenty years, he would wait for me.

Instead, I had a string of relationships with men who treated me badly in one way or another, which took its toll on my health. Some were insecure and belittled me because they were threatened or jealous. Others were pathological flirts with commitment issues. One was still in love with his ex-girlfriend.

I ran into Charlie every few years, and he always had a big smile. My heart would swell, and I would question myself: *Why can't I love someone like him? Why do I always choose men who hurt me?*

After nearly losing my mom to a brain hemorrhage and breaking up with a man who always put his work first, I spent two months alone on a Greek island. It was a time to examine my life in a new way. Something had changed in me, and I began to think about what was really important. Suddenly, Charlie was on my mind, and soon all I could think about was him.

I must have been on his mind, too, because one hot afternoon I walked up the dirt road to the nearby village to check my messages from a pay phone, and there was a message from him!

This had to be a sign. I knew that on my return I would see him, and I finally felt ready to meet him in the place he had always been—a place of love.

When I got home, I called and left him a message. And then I waited for him to call me back, and for our life to begin together. But days passed with no word from him, and then weeks.

Finally, a mutual friend told me the news. He was in the hospital with cancer.

I went to see Charlie in the hospital. He had a tube in his throat and couldn't talk, but he was smiling and light. Charlie's friend, who was watching over the sickbed, seemed concerned to see a face she didn't recognize, but Charlie wrote on his notepad, "It's okay. She's like family."

I said, "I love you, Charlie," and we held each other's gaze. Then a nurse ushered me out for a shift change.

I wanted to go back and see him again. But when I tried to return, I wasn't allowed back in the room. His family didn't want me to be near him. To them, I was just the girl who broke Charlie's heart, and I was sent away.

I spent the next two weeks hearing of Charlie's decline from friends. I couldn't eat or sleep. He visited me in dreams, every night becoming less human and more angel, imparting wisdom that seemed to come from another realm.

I never saw him again.

When I lost Charlie, I thought I had also lost the hope for romantic love. The wound was so deep that it took years to heal. But the healing didn't truly take hold until I took my first dose of a homeopathic remedy called Ignatia. Ignatia amara is a homeopathic remedy for emotional shock and grief. It is a powerful remedy for people who feel so much sorrow they are afraid to let it out for fear it will never end—and so they suffer from suppressing their emotions.

When I took Ignatia, I felt everything that was not *me* lift away. All the bitterness, heaviness, and hopelessness faded, replaced by existential bliss. It was an exciting and powerful feeling.

Suddenly, I thought, *I remember the last time I felt this way*. I was four years old the last time I had felt truly happy and relaxed, the last time I felt a real openness and love for everyone I encountered. That was before my parents started fighting, before the alcoholism and separation, the abandonment and the chronic disappointment of a shattered family. I had been returned to my true nature, the way I had come into the world.

And then I realized that I had not just been heartbroken since Charlie died—I had been heartbroken since childhood. That was why I couldn't accept the kind of love Charlie had given me—I could only be with people who were going to continue to break my heart because that was the emotional place I had been stuck in for all those years.

After that, heartbreak became less appealing. I still dip my toe in the waters of sadness now and again—I still love melancholy music and sad movies—but heartbreak is not where I reside anymore. My home in this world is happy, light, and free.

Now, to find a man like Charlie to share it with me!

HEART-HEALING MEDITATION: GROUNDING CORD MEDITATION

A grounding cord meditation connects you to a slower, calming Earth energy. By visualizing a grounding cord that runs from your sacrum to the ground, like the roots from a tree, you can use your mind and imagination productively to release pain and deep emotions. Imagine any old thought patterns that do not serve you are being released through the grounding cord and allow the Mother Earth energy to rise up and cleanse you of unwanted emotions.

Find a tree and sit beside it, with your sacrum (tailbone) at the base of the tree. Sit up with a straight spine, leaning against the tree. Feel the power and the life force of the tree. As you close your eyes, feel your life force and the life force of the tree connecting. As you imagine the roots of the tree grounding deeply into the earth, experience yourself following the roots deep down and grounding firmly into the center of the Earth.

You may also do this practice from the comfort of your own home. If you do so, I suggest that you sit in a chair, with both feet flat on the ground and your spine straight. Soften your breath and feel all the support of the ground beneath you and/or the tree beside you. Breathe for 15–20 minutes. When you are done, give thanks and open your eyes.

LOVE NOTES: THE GRATITUDE LIST

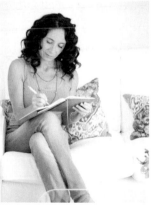

More and more these days we hear that happiness is increased by the expression of gratitude. There is a theory that what you focus on expands, and that if you list the things you are grateful for, your spirits will be elevated. It can be difficult to see the positive when the things you love are lost. However, I am here to say from experience that it really does work. But don't just take my word for it. Create a gratitude list daily, and see what happens to you. It sounds pretty easy, but at first it can be a real struggle to identify the joy when you are feeling down. But try anyway: simply write ten things you are grateful for. Though these can be broad, try to be specific, especially to see the things around you that you may take for granted.

Your daily gratitude list may look something like this:

I am grateful for:

- The ability to take deep breaths
- The moon hanging in the sky
- My legs—they get me where I need to go
- This heavyheartedness, for strengthening my self-nurture
- The miracle of life
- The ability to feel deep sadness and the heights of joy
- Being human
- Animals
- Crushed ice
- Friends I can call

ADVANCED MOVE: WRITE A HEARTBREAK GRATITUDE LIST

Put what pains you at the top of the list. What if the very thing that is your greatest challenge is actually your greatest gift? I know for a fact that the breakup that crushed me and sent me to my knees was a blessing. I am incredibly grateful for that relationship, but I had an even better one after that, and am sure that my next one will be even more appropriate for me. It may be hard at first for you to see a place for gratitude in your despair, but as you grow down you may be surprised at what you find. Here are just a few things I was grateful for:

- I get to heal and find my strength in adversity
- I don't need to check in with anyone when I make a plan
- I have the ability to feel deeply
- I can develop compassion for others who have the same pain
- There's the possibility that I get to fall in love again
- I get to learn about myself and what soothes me
- I can spread out in the bed and use *all* the pillows

- I don't have to clean up after someone else

- I get Girlfriend Time

- I'll encounter surprises I can't even imagine yet

RITUAL: A GIFT OF LOVE

You deserve love. Taking an action like buying yourself a bouquet of flowers can give you a sense that you are loved. By *you*. When I went through a particularly difficult emotional period, I lived in a guesthouse that had rose bushes everywhere. Each week I cut myself fresh roses. Roses have the highest vibration of all flowers. The scent of the roses had healing properties for me. I could feel my heart being healed and my energies being lifted with every inhalation.

This week: drink rose tea and buy or make a floral bouquet with healing properties, as described on page 184.

STRENGTH FOR THE SOUL: FLOWERS THAT HEAL

According to Alexis Smart, "Dr. Edward Bach's flower remedy system was discovered in the 1930s. Dissatisfied with the medicine of the day, Dr. Bach felt that only the body was treated, while the patient's emotional state was neglected. He discovered that the essences of blossoming flowers, when taken internally, had a profoundly positive effect on the emotions of the patients, and once they felt happy, their illnesses would miraculously resolve."

Alexis's story (page 178) is a testament to the profound effect of using flower remedies to soothe the melancholy that may come with lost love. She shares that the subtle and gentle nature of the essences are vibrational and may also be used with other healing modalities or medicines. Another bonus: there is no danger in taking the wrong ones.

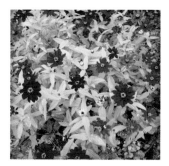

Alexis recommends making your own custom blend, saying, "It's fun to play alchemist and let your intuition guide you." Try her DIY recipe on the next page using the Bach flower remedies listed. The Bach line can be found at most health food stores or at a favorite online resource, www.fesflowers.com. If you feel intimidated making it yourself, try one of Alexis's custom blends, available at www.AlexisSmart. com. The WholeHearted blend heals recent sorrow, and InLove helps to attract healthy relationships.

ALEXIS SMART'S DIY FLOWER REMEDY INSTRUCTIONS:

This is Alexis's simple broad-spectrum flower remedy recipe for when you feel down:

- Rescue Remedy*
- Sweet Chestnut
- Honeysuckle
- Star of Bethlehem

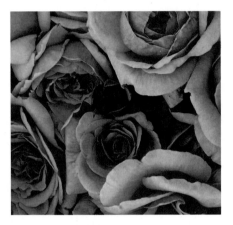

Put 4 drops of each essence into a 1-ounce dosage bottle of spring water and shake gently. From this bottle, take 4 drops under the tongue 4 times a day. The effects are cumulative and best results will be felt at about the third week. You may also add drops to a glass of water and sip throughout the day.

Or, if you like you can create your own remedy:

Combine up to four of the flower essences from the list on the next page. But no matter what your formula, include Star of Bethlehem. Any unhealed shock or trauma can prevent the other remedies from being effective, but Star of Bethlehem, according to the www.BachFlower.org website, "neutralizes any form of energetic trauma, integrates the actions of the other . . . flower remedies, and quickly restores the body's self-healing abilities."

---

* Made by BachFlower, the Rescue Remedy—also called the five-flower formula—is a signature blend of flowers formulated to reduce stress and anxiety.

FLOWER ESSENCE	REMEDY FOR . . .
Centaury	Standing up for yourself, saying "no," breaking free of dominant personalities
Chicory	Abandonment, self-pity
Holly	Jealousy, feelings of hatred, revenge
Heather	Self-absorption, loneliness, neediness
Honeysuckle	Nostalgia, living in the past
Pine	Guilt and self-blame, feeling undeserving of love
Star of Bethlehem	Grief, sadness, emotional shock (past and present)
Sweet chestnut	Despair and hopelessness, intense anguish
Walnut	Difficulty accepting change
Willow	Bitterness, resentment, victim mentality, self-pity

HEART FACT A recent study at Rutgers, the State University of New Jersey, showed that flowers can have a positive impact on people's moods, increasing feelings such as happiness, surprise, and enjoyment.

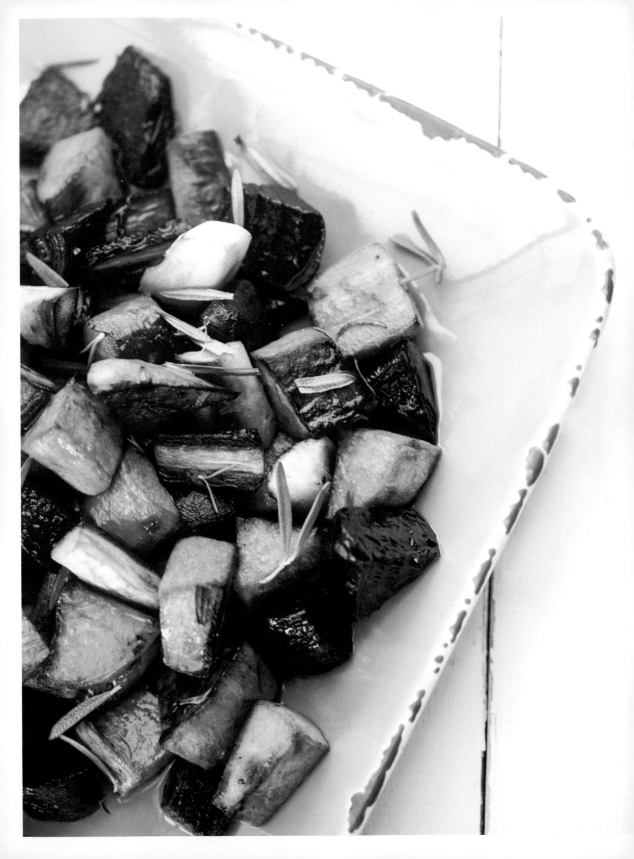

ROASTED ROOT VEGETABLES

Serves 2—4

This easy-to-make heart-healthy recipe comes from the root . . . literally. The heartiness of this root vegetable dish will ground you with simplicity and earthiness—while providing you with high levels of the vitamins and minerals these vegetables absorb from the soil. Beets have anti-inflammatory properties, carrots are known to prevent cardiovascular disease, yams are antioxidants, and parsnips are an excellent source of vitamin C, folate, and manganese.

2 CARROTS

2 BEETS

1 YAM

1 PARSNIP

OLIVE OIL (TO COAT VEGETABLES)

FRESH ROSEMARY

2 TABLESPOONS
    BALSAMIC VINEGAR

SALT AND PEPPER

Heat oven to 450°F.

Chop vegetables into 1-inch squares. Combine in a bowl and coat with the olive oil, rosemary, and vinegar.

Roast the veggies until browned. (I like them extra crispy.) Season to taste with salt and pepper.

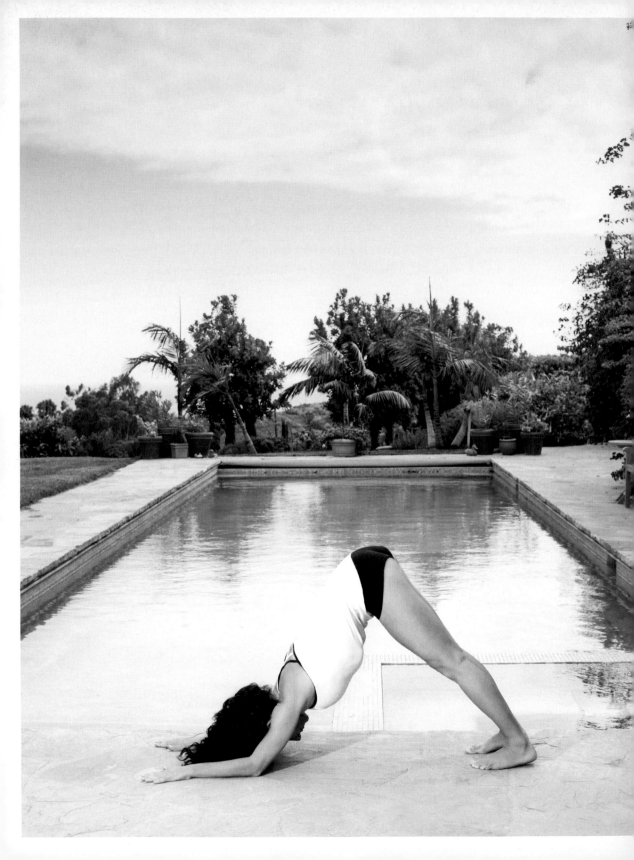

WEEK 3

Talk Your Walk

In this chapter you'll learn how to "talk your walk." I know what you're thinking: what the heck does that mean? Allow me to explain. When you walk, you put one foot in front of the other, and you have faith that each step will lead you to the next in a way that keeps you moving forward. Now, imagine you're walking on a bumpy, unpaved road—like life. Presence in the moment is crucial to be surefooted, yet most of us have been walking for so long we do it unconsciously, without intention, presence, or direction. Our unconscious thoughts are directing our walk.

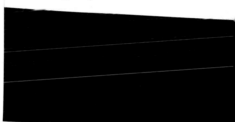

Taking this notion a little further, consider this: out of your unconcious mind come the words you speak. Then those thoughts become your actions—or your walk. If you stick with this framework, you're haphazardly allowing your unharnessed thoughts to chart your path. But that's not the only way to live. To help direct where your steps take you, you must gain presence of mind and rethink habitual directions you may unconsciously give yourself *before* taking action. Then declare where you are going. This is talking your walk.

Your words, whether thought or spoken, are like a magical spell or an incantation. You may not be in control of your first thought, but you are in control of your second thought. The way that you frame and spin your first thought matters. Reframing the way you talk about yourself, others, and your circumstances has a direct effect upon the world you walk through. Words can scar; words can be used as a weapon to hurt others. They can also be used as a salve and a medicine. Sometimes the words you use can be like a corrective brace, harnessing the thoughts you think and altering your view.

This week we'll explore how to use words to create your reality and how to frame your story in ways that reflect your faith and bring you comfort and strength. If that doesn't sound like fun, consider this: the beauty of reframing loss, and with talking your walk, is you have choices. You get to rediscover and reinvent yourself. You are not the same person that you were prior to the heartbreak. There are new layers to be found.

This is just like a yoga practice. Within a framework is the discovery of unexplored places in your body and mind you have not accessed in a while, which requires a little bit of patience, practice, and curiosity. You also have new muscles that have strengthened and abilities that were not available prior to your circumstance. You now get to bring those muscles you developed back to the practice on your mat to see what this allows you in yoga—and in life.

worrier. I remember, even then, future tripping that my mom [...] y to pick me up from school—and then what would I do? I felt insecure. Faith was something that I needed to train myself to feel; it didn't set in by itself. I needed proof. In time, life's circumstances and the experiences I'd been through provided me with that proof. Faith is the key to feeling taken care of and truly loved. By definition faith requires belief that something out there in the universe has got your back. I usually require experience from the universe to back that up. You can rely on that force for an outcome that is correct. Life itself has offered me experiences that were devastating in the moment, but turned out to lead me down a path that was far better than I had ever imagined. All the same, my "setting" is not naturally calibrated to be optimistic and in faith.

I know that even those who have a positive mind-set are not exempt from feeling the depths of despair and powerlessness that life inevitably brings. It's how they handle it that offers a different outcome. My mother, who is a very optimistic person, is a great example of this. Watching her go through a cataclysmic break up with my dad, and it being the first divorce I ever witnessed, I remember the depth of emotion that she felt. It was not easy to witness her sorrowful and animalistic mourning process.

In retrospect, the fact that she allowed me to see her grieving process uncensored was incredibly generous. She took her space and time with the emptiness and loss. This upheaval catapulted her into unknown terrain. After all, my mother had gone straight from living with her parents to marrying my father at age nineteen; at age twenty she birthed me, and by age twenty-two she was the mother of two and the head of the household. All she knew was the life she had as a wife and mother. She had no identity of her own to return to, and no sense of her place in the external world. Not only that, but it was a big surprise to her that my father cheated on her, for she had never imagined that.

Her entire world was being recalibrated. Her truth was turned upside down. Through her devastation, I did not know what to do for her. In her process she realigned with herself. She did not accept a lot of outside advice or ideas because she didn't want to reinforce the negativity of the "story." She knew her own true north and inner compass would guide her.

Within a year and a half, my mother had fully grieved. She became a personal assistant to make ends meet. It was while she was working as an assistant that one of the painters on the job, Stephen, developed a crush on my beautiful mother. The only issue was that he was fourteen years her junior, and he had to win her over, which he did. Once he spent the night, he never left her side—and that was thirty years ago. They are best friends to this day, and people in their apartment building still call them "the honeymoon couple."

My mother's experience showed me that, while there are no guarantees of the outcome, you can still choose to be happy and look on the bright side. She continues to talk that walk in the face of challenges regarding Stephen's health. Adding to his back surgeries and problems throughout the years, which invariably cause hardship for him and those around him, several months ago he had two strokes. The initial stroke, although serious, had no visible effects, yet they did find two bleeds in his brain and identified that he needed two procedures to stop them. But what's worse is they found a third bleed, a ticking time bomb in his head. As I write this, he is in the hospital post brain surgery.

Initially, when they found this out, my mother said, in her usual positive tone, "Well, it was a difficult morning . . ." Usually when I ask how things are she says: "We are doing okay, considering how we are doing." Or she points out what they *do* still have. "We're still here, able to communicate with each other. He can move around." Just last night, she revealed that Stephen has never felt this level of love, support, and connection with others. The way my mother talks about the situation allows her to focus on the positive and have the best possible experience in the moment, which is quite an education for me. I have learned to join the choir and chime in, with comments like: "He has had a lot of love with his two brothers and from his parents. It's been a real healing for their family." I'm learning.

This way of framing loss by focusing on true blessings is a magical direction to take. The words we choose and the way we tell our story has a huge effect on our outcomes. Life asks for evidence of our faith, and times like these are when we are really put to the test. Can we have faith and trust that the universe wants for us what is best and will offer tremendous gifts?

I aim to help you answer "yes" to this question this week as we work together to begin to frame your story in ways that reflect your faith. I am not saying to sugarcoat or deny your feelings, but to find a way to talk that projects the best possible outcome. The gratitude list from the previous week should ignite a feeling of hope—and, out of that hope, a wellspring of the faith I'm referring to.

Journaling, one of the exercises this week, is a wonderful way to find and express your feelings. It's also key to bringing consciousness to your talk and is a way of reconnecting with the heart. When you put pen to paper the universe can come right in to express itself, your words flowing from your heart down your arm into your pen. It is through your heart that you access your love and become closer to harmonizing with the vibration of your highest self. Speak with love, for your words have power. Love with your words and your thoughts. As you come to harness the mind, the fluctuations of your thoughts will no longer disturb you. It takes practice, but talking your walk leads to a very high level of being.

"Be careful of your thoughts, for your thoughts become your words.
Be careful of your words, for your words become your actions.
Be careful of your actions, for your actions become your habits.
Be careful of your habits, for your habits become your character.
Be careful of your character, for your character becomes your destiny."
—Chinese proverb

SELF-LOVE CHECKLIST

YOGALOSOPHY FOR INNER STRENGTH program

- ☐ **Sunday:** Be Happy Yoga
- ☐ **Monday:** Back-to-Basics Yoga
- ☐ **Tuesday:** Cardio
- ☐ **Wednesday:** Bounce Back! Yoga
- ☐ **Thursday:** Day Off
- ☐ **Friday:** Let Go Yoga
- ☐ **Saturday:** Get Strong Yogalosophy
- ☐ **Heart-Opening Pose:** Dolphin
- ☐ **Love Movement:** Neighborhood Walk
- ☐ **Heart-Healing Meditation:** Mantra
- ☐ **Love Notes:** Write a Love Note to Yourself
- ☐ **Ritual:** Make a Book About You
- ☐ **Strength for the Soul:** 10 Things I Love About Me

MANTRA

I am willing to be open to think and speak positively about my circumstances. I have faith that step by step, I will know where to go.

TRACK OF THE WEEK

"Stranger in a Strange Land" by Leon Russell, "Be Here Now" by Ray LaMontagne, or "Hell Yeah" by Ani DiFranco

- Start on your hands and knees, with your knees directly below your hips. Place your forearms on the mat, shoulder-width apart. Align your wrists and elbows. Press your palms down with fingers spread wide.

- Tuck your toes under, inhale, and lift your hips on the exhale. Keep your knees slightly bent as you aim your sit bones toward the ceiling. Soften your heart toward the floor.

- Slowly straighten your legs, allowing your heels to sink as your legs straighten. Actively press your forearms and palms into the mat. Hang your head between your shoulders, allowing the traction to create a deep shoulder stretch. (Keep your knees bent if your back is rounding.) Lengthen your tailbone away from your pelvis as you extend your sternum toward the floor.

- Hold for 5–10 breaths. This posture works the back and helps to strengthen and free the shoulders. This serves not only as a heart-opening pose but also as an inversion, which reverses your blood flow and calms the nervous system.

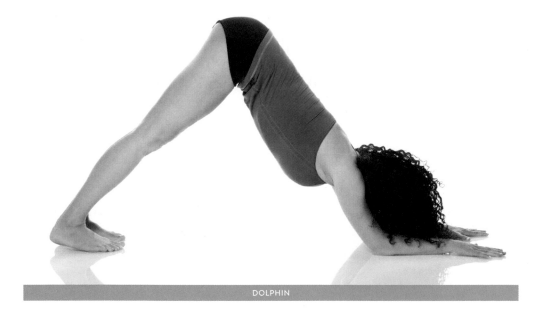

DOLPHIN

LOVE MOVEMENT: NEIGHBORHOOD WALK

Every day this week take a walk in your neighborhood to connect with your surroundings. Do so in as present a way as possible. This is not a rote exercise, but an exercise in being present moment to moment. Say hello to people and make eye contact. You are not alone. It's important to get out of the self and to remember that you are connected to other human beings. Love is everywhere. A neighborhood walk can change your day and immediately make you feel less alone. Notice what's happening in your neighborhood: the little animals walking their humans, people preparing their dinners, the self-discipline of joggers, elderly couples walking together hand in hand. There are so many beautiful human treasures all around us that daily bless us with the love of the universe. Take them in.

LINDA'S STORY

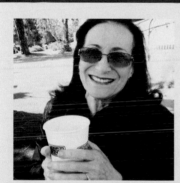

My first guest contributor this week is my very own mother, Linda Ingber. What I can tell you is that she is a kind woman with a lot of integrity; she is positive and incredibly entertaining. Her foundation of loss gave her an indomitable spirit that always blows my mind. After first being a mom to my brother and me, she has tutored children privately in Los Angeles for eighteen years. Here is a little taste of her.

• • •

Linda

I was born in a displaced persons camp in post–World War II Germany. These camps were created for the survivors of WWII who were rendered homeless as a result of the Holocaust.

It was far from glamorous living in army barracks surrounded by barbed wire fences, but it was my home. We were a tight-knit family that consisted of my mother, father, maternal grandmother, older brother, and me. For nearly four years we lived in the camps, along with many other refugees who had also been displaced; this was our community.

In 1951, we were invited by the U.S. government to come and live in the United States. In February of that year we boarded a U.S. Navy ship and crossed the stormy Atlantic to the eastern shores of America. My protests to turn around and go home were to no avail. When we arrived, it felt like we had traveled to a distant galaxy where no one was like us or spoke our language. Life, as I knew it, was over. We were strangers in a strange land.

Everything was different in this new place: weird language, different clothing, new food, new customs, and an entirely different lifestyle; it was total culture shock. When it was time for me to enroll in school, our American cousin insisted that my name be changed. "Chava Luba" was no longer suitable in this new land, so I was renamed. I would henceforth be known as: Linda.

To complicate matters further, my parents were unable to offer me any help with my homework. They had their own struggles with the English language to contend with. I was on my own. It was sink or swim and, fortunately, I became a good "swimmer." I not only thought that school was a great place, I took my studies seriously and proved to be a good student.

Many years have passed since that time. As I reflect on my life's path, it's clear that the traumatic departure from my first home actually proved to be invaluable. As fate would have it, Chava Luba, the immigrant girl, grew up to be a teacher of the English language.

Over time, I have had the pleasure and privilege of teaching a large number of students, some of whom have come from homes where English was not spoken. Imagine their surprise when I shared that English was not my first language either. I was living proof that they, too, could do it.

As a result of departing from Germany so many years ago, I gained a deeper understanding of how to adapt to new situations and assimilate successfully. I also grew up to do something that I love, which is to teach. Ultimately, what tickles me the most, to this day, is the irony that I came all the way from Germany to teach English in America.

JENNI'S STORY

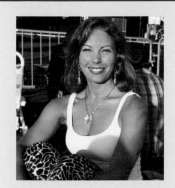

My other guest contributor for this week is Jenni Anspach, who was instrumental in helping me put this book together. You can find her recipes on pages 201 and 203. A photographer, yogini, chef, writer, and right- *and* left-hand woman, Jenni knows all about framing her experiences. That means that even if you're as far away from detaching from your story as I can be, Jenni can show you how!

• • •

Jenni

Though hindsight is 20/20 and lessons from heartbreak tend to present themselves later on, at the time most of us would never *choose* to be heartbroken. Most people try to "get over it" to somehow extinguish any positive feelings they have for the other person. Others dwell on a past relationship so much that they enter a kind of limbo state, never allowing their heart to reopen. I believe that genuine love never has to be suppressed or possessed . . . although it may have to change form. That *is* a choice—it's an intention.

There's a saying in Hawaiian Huna philosophy, "Bless that which you want." From my experience, the most healing thing in moving through heartbreak has not been to try to escape from the pain, but instead to bless the other person on their journey. And that includes any newfound happiness they may be experiencing. (Believe me, growing into being able to *truly* do this has been a process!)

People I've loved in the past I continue to love to this day, just in a different way. When I've loved a person, it meant that I loved *them*: not for who they were when I was with them, but for who they were on their own. So what was I to do with that love when it ended? Perhaps you can relate—when you're in love with somebody, you want their happiness with your whole heart and soul and every fiber of your being, and when you split up, suddenly their happiness becomes your anguish and resentment.

Well, you can channel the love that still exists. You can transmute the romantic love that you felt into an even more expansive love. You can wish them the same immense joy in life, even though it may not include you anymore. This heals you by resolving the perceived conflict of "I still love them" and "I'm not with them." It may sound idealistic, or naive, maybe even impossible, and it doesn't mean it may not still hurt from time to time—but if you can wish happiness for the same person that deserved so much of your heart, as they travel the path that was meant for them, you will actually be blessing your own path and creating space for the one that was meant for you.

HEART-HEALING MEDITATION: MANTRA

A mantra is generally a word that represents a name for God or the Divine. You don't have to believe in God, like a bearded man watching over you, or gods like in Greek mythology. However, there certainly is a force in the world that keeps the sun rising and setting and breathes waves into the ocean. It's that force of nature that beats your heart and breathes life into you without your own effort. You can rely on that life force. The word *"yam"* is the sound that resonates with the heart. The mantra is like a code that allows you to download the sacred intelligence of the fourth chakra energy center that I highlighted in Week 1. As you chant *yam,* sense the vibration and consciousness of the sound as it resonates with your heart. Open up and receive the love, compassion, and joy that resides within you. Spend 2 to 5 minutes chanting *yam* at your own volume and pace each day this week, and notice the way you feel. (If you are resistant to speaking *yam* you may replace it with "yes.")

LOVE NOTES: WRITE A LOVE NOTE TO YOURSELF

This week, write a love note to yourself. Tell yourself all of the wonderful things that you need to hear, and remind yourself how much you love you.

RITUAL: MAKE A BOOK ABOUT *YOU*

When I was a child, I got this great Dr. Seuss book, *My Book About Me.* It was a yellow book. (Coincidentally, yellow relates to the third chakra, which is connected to the self and the identity. It's also directly related to the mind and thinking.) The book was a questionnaire all about what you like. As a girl in school I carried this into my friendships, sending the same questions to my best friends to fill out in order to get to know them better. It's time to get to know yourself again with a "what I like" inventory, a book that will be all about you. So ask yourself questions like: What is my favorite flower? Animal? Scent? What is my go-to comfort food? What movie makes me laugh? When

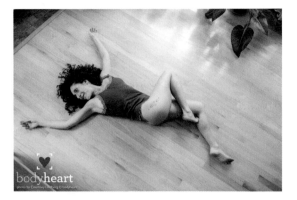

I get angry I like to: ___. When I feel sad, the best thing I can do for myself is: ___. I feel powerful when: ___. If I had a superpower it would be: ___. And so forth. Be creative!

You will need:

- Various kinds of paper (thick, thin, colored, white)
- A printed photograph of yourself
- Colorful markers, pens, pencils, etc.
- Adhesives like a stapler, glue, tape, etc.
- Glitter, stickers, buttons—whatever else you would like to use for your book

See the questions above for ideas. You can include things like your favorite dinner entrée, favorite color, favorite flower, favorite clothing, favorite scent, etc.

STRENGTH FOR THE SOUL: TEN THINGS I LOVE ABOUT ME!

Write a daily list of ten things you love about yourself. This is not about the fact that you have great friends—it's that you *are* a great friend. This is not about the work you do—it's about the *way* you do your work. This is about the real you. I know that this exercise can be a challenge, but that's because it's new behavior. You are loveable just because you are here. Be that voice for yourself all week.

HEART FACT
Did you know that the first heart cell starts to beat as early as four weeks from conception?

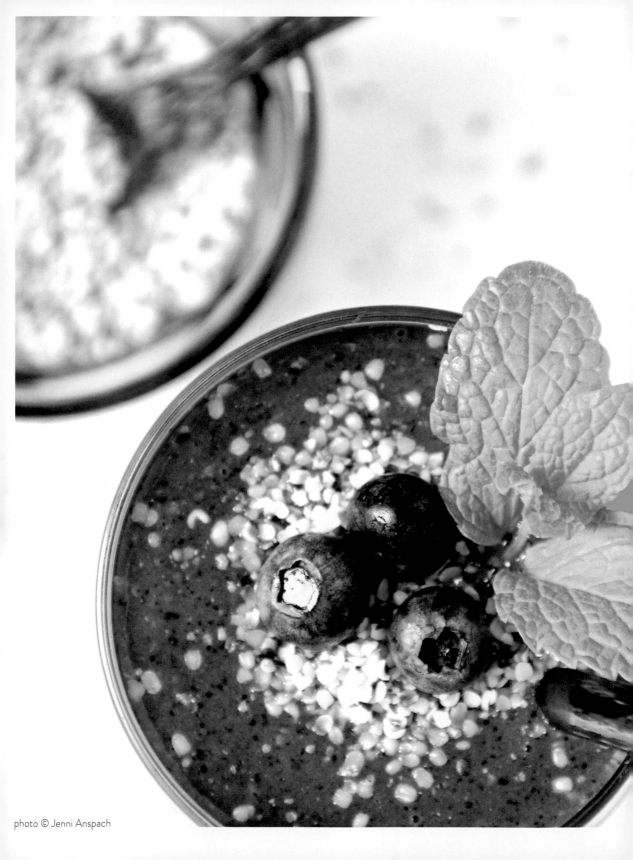

CHOCOLATE BLUEBERRY DAYDREAM SMOOTHIE

Serves 1—2

Cacao opens capillaries, nourishes the nervous system, promotes endorphins, and aids metabolism. Maca boosts libido and increases stamina, and is good for hormonal and emotional balance. Hempseed has omega-3s, minerals, and protein. Blueberries are rich in antioxidants, and bananas are a great source of potassium (a mineral electrolyte that helps maintain the flow of the electricity that keeps your heart beating!).

2 HANDFULS FRESH BLUEBERRIES

1 LARGE BANANA (OR 1¹/₂ SMALL)

1 CUP UNSWEETENED ALMOND MILK

1 TABLESPOON CACAO POWDER

1 TEASPOON RAW CACAO NIBS

1 TEASPOON HEMPSEED

1 TABLESPOON MACA POWDER

1 TEASPOON HONEY (IF DESIRED)

Put all ingredients in a blender.

Blend. Drink. Dream . . .

Recipe by Jenni Anspach

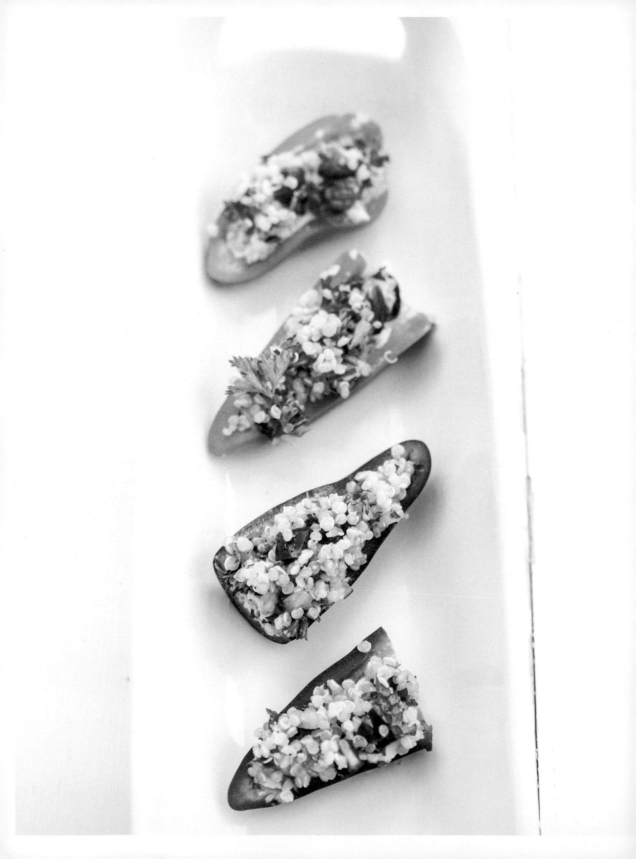

RAW STUFFED MINI PEPPERS WITH HUMMUS AND QUINOA TABOULEH

Serves 2—4

The quinoa tabouleh on its own makes a great healthy side dish; the stuffed mini peppers create a perfect snack for one or a fun appetizer for a get-together. (Choose the largest mini bell peppers you can, as you will be filling them.) Quinoa is a great plant-based protein—it's actually considered a "complete protein," as it has high amounts of all the essential amino acids we need in our diet.

1/2 CUP WHITE QUINOA

1 CUP WATER

1 CUP PARSLEY, FINELY CHOPPED*

1/3 CUP MINT, FINELY CHOPPED*

12 CHERRY TOMATOES, FINELY DICED*

1/4 CUP RED ONION, FINELY DICED*

1 TO 2 TABLESPOONS OLIVE OIL

1 TABLESPOON FRESH LEMON JUICE

SALT AND PEPPER

10–12 MINI MULTICOLORED BELL PEPPERS

1 10-OUNCE CONTAINER OF HUMMUS

Since the bell peppers are mini, you'll want to chop and dice as finely as possible.

To make the tabouleh, cook the quinoa and allow it to cool. (Cooking 1/2 cup of quinoa in 1 cup of water should yield at least 1 cup cooked.) In a large bowl combine the cooled quinoa, parsley, mint, cherry tomatoes, and red onion. Drizzle the olive oil and lemon juice over the top, then add salt and pepper to taste.

Slice the tops off the mini bell peppers and cut them in half lengthwise. Scoop out any seeds. Using a spoon or a piping bag, put a layer of hummus in the bottoms of the peppers. Top each pepper with a spoonful of tabouleh, which should stick well to the hummus. Enjoy!

Recipe by Jenni Anspach

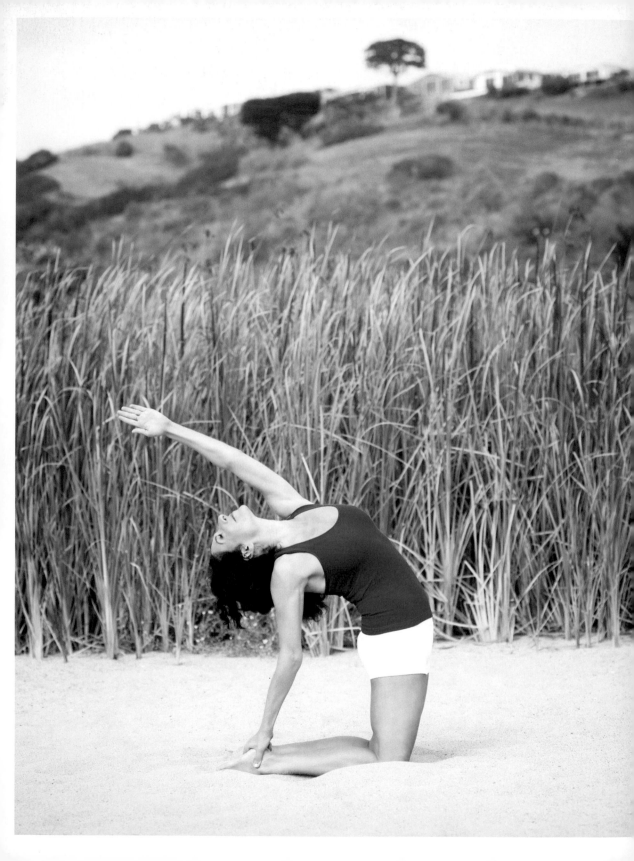

WEEK 4

Be Your Own Mother

The root of the word "courage" is derived from the Latin word *cor*, meaning heart. The connection is meaningful here: it takes courage to dive into your emotions, especially when they're not happy ones. It can feel like you're blindly leaping headfirst into a vast ocean—knowing that it's only once you jump in that you'll face what's beneath the surface. I tell you this now because this week we're going to plunge into our pasts and our "mother wound"—the ones we got from our mom (or lack thereof) that scarred us and formed some of our thinking and behavior. And then we're going to explore healing those wounds by learning how to self-mother, giving ourselves the nurturing, restorative benefits that good mothering brings.

"The mother understands the heart of the child; she pours her love into the child, teaches him or her the positive lessons of life, and corrects the child's mistakes."

—AMMA, FROM THE AWAKENING OF UNIVERSAL MOTHERHOOD: GENEVA SPEECH

I am not a mother. The oddity does not escape me that when I see a mother and her children my tendency is to relate more to the child's point of view. Even if you are not a mother yourself, you have some experience with "mothering." Becoming a mother takes a huge amount of courage. When I conjure a picture of idyllic mothering, it arouses a feeling of the elder having a direct bond and almost psychic connection with this innocent extension of the self. The mother intuitively feels what the child feels and, as the experienced being, knows the needs of the child—while having developed

205

the tools and the maturity to resolve and contain the needs of the child. Is this the type of mothering you got? Me neither.

Many people have a wound or a sense of loss around their own mothers or mothering. The idyllic mother is a joyful nurturer, feeding the child physically and emotionally in order for the child to grow and develop. She is a protector who guards the child from abuse and outside threats so that the child can feel trusting and safe. She is an empowerer, who encourages self-confidence by allowing independence and encourages self-reliance by providing discipline and guidelines. The mother is the initiator, providing a sense of meaning and purpose to the child's life as part of the world at large. It is a tall order to ask one source to provide all of this, and yet this is intrinsically what each of us needs. It is so common for us to feel we didn't get it that there's actually a term for the form of loss that emerges as a result: the "mother wound."

The very first wound of the heart, for all human beings, is the mother wound. Society sets us up for this archetypal heartbreak. The mother/child bond is the one bond we make *to* break. Recognizing that your mother could not provide you with all that you need, and may have even directed subconscious anger toward you, gives you an opportunity to grieve. You don't have to take care of your mother by staying meek. There are many expressions of the mother wound. According to an article by expert Bethany Webster: without healing this wound you may have weakened boundaries, feel unsafe to voice your truth, or be unable to make a breakthrough. This may manifest in relationships where you play the emotional caretaker role, have a high tolerance for being mistreated, are rigid, or develop eating disorders and addictions. When you take the time to heal from the mother wound, you become more emotionally skilled and have a true sense of how to mother yourself. You have a deep, felt compassion for yourself and others and trust life.

✖ MY STORY

I love my mom, and she is awesome to be around. Completely entertaining, fun, and loyal. But my mother was a child herself when she had me. At just twenty years old she was presented with a being to care for and pour love into. We can only love others to the extent we love ourselves, and my mother had a lot of experience in her bones, but not with herself alone. She was raised in essence by her grandmother, since her mother was put to work in the coal mines of Russia. Her mother, my maternal grandmother, was blessed with two children: the elder, my uncle, born in a cabin in Siberia; and then Chava Luba, my mom, born in a displaced person's camp in Germany after the war. When they all journeyed to the United States on a boat, my mother was plunged into a world she had never known, with an entirely new language to learn. She and her brother were put to task, as they would go to school to learn English and return with lessons that they would teach their own parents. My mother was a born teacher; in fact she found this to be her calling in her later years and became a teacher at age fifty. She still teaches to this day.

When my mother was ten her primary caregiver, her grandmother, passed away, and she was left in charge of cooking and cleaning while her parents worked to make ends meet. Seven years later, she met my father and they dated, eventually married, and then there I was. I know that my mother's situation was not uncommon in 1968. After all, women were raised under the assumption that they would marry and then become mothers themselves. It was a given. I see my generation as the first in which we were actually raised to have choices. The expectations on women have shifted considerably and no longer perpetuate a conveyor belt of the same old models, varieties, or patterns. When I look back, I so admire these women who blossomed under the canopy of family, and discovered themselves through the familial dynamics.

The dynamics in my home were hot. As my parents struggled to find their adult identities, arguing and miscommunication were as common as breakfast. There I was, a quite sensitive little unit, and I did not feel safe. The emotional storms that surrounded me were drowning me and I learned to stay undercover, to be "good," and not to verbalize my fear or my deep loneliness. I had to survive and make the best of things, which I did. It was easier for my mother if I didn't lay upon her my own depths of despair, which would have just added to the turmoil that surrounded us all. I must have stopped wanting to have needs at a preverbal age. I may have even thought, *This is my fault*. Who knows? What I do know is that, for whatever reason, I learned not to talk about my true feelings and not to trust the way I felt. I even became numb to my actual feelings. I was praised for being well behaved, for coloring inside the lines, and for being helpful. Underneath it all, the war between my parents and in my family of origin frightened me, and had me shaking in my booties.

On the flip side, my childhood could be extremely fun at times. My mother was an entertaining teacher and best friend, so the bonuses of laughter, puppet shows, and creative projects were great. But somehow I was still lost. The emotional rollercoaster ride of my childhood had me in a state of shock, and since I never knew what was coming next, I simply held on until the next wave. Thankfully, my creativity always saved me. I could channel that nebulous intensity, nervous energy, and depth into my multiple creative projects, for which I was praised. I had a knack for creative expression. This was where I found the empowerment and sense of initiation into a bigger world.

By the age of eleven, I got the acting bug. This new passion gave me a container to feel my emotions fully with total acceptance. This was a gearshift for me, and I found that when I was hiding behind a character I was able to fully dive in to feeling and experience the full range of my human emotions. What liberation! Only, it opened up the emotional floodgates for me. Once I was able to access myself, there was no turning back.

One of the best things about self-exploration in acting is that you are given accolades for finding your truth. Your raw, human, and even unattractive parts are pulled to the surface, recognized, seen, and celebrated. At last: a place to *feel* fully. When I was masked in character, I could allow my fierceness to rage. My sorrow was so beautifully contained by the well-written words of our greatest playwrights. My sexuality was celebrated behind the safety of an audience. So this was the first step for me: allowing myself to feel and to be expressed. At first it was easier to try this in a scene instead of in my real life. Later, I explored living a "real life" by becoming a fitness instructor. It was there that I furthered my healing of the "mother wound"—by using my voice as a tool for nurturing, empowering, protecting, and initiating my students.

Spinning classes and yoga, or any exercise regime, is a place to channel all of the emotional energy that you feel—to a positive effect. You can actually feel your emotions fueling you as you connect to the motivational speaking of a teacher paired with the music that accompanies the movement. It ignites the very essence of human desire via the emotional energy that is stored in our bodies. Perhaps one of the most difficult parts of loss is the dull and listless feeling, the blanket of depression that can flatten you. Bottom line: emotions speak in the language of the body. It's good to get your feet wet and get involved in that conversation. I am not saying you have to jump up and get moving the moment you are down, but I do know that physical activity is one of the fastest and most immediate ways to move out of the low and bring your energy and vibration up. Still, at moments, you must simply allow for your need to feel sad.

My mother once gave me advice about getting over a broken heart. She said it would pass if I gave it time. She told me that every day I would feel a little better, just like when I was getting over the flu. I held on to that image. After all, I'd seen her go through it and she was just fine. I liked hearing her words. However, I found that relying on my mother somehow diminished me. When I spoke with her, I would feel better temporarily, but then I would get weaker. I knew that I had to find that voice in myself. It was this awareness that led me to look within for the self-mothering I needed.

Self-discovery is simply a deepening of the intimacy with self. Today, I understand myself because I know more than ever that I can trust how I feel. Although feelings are not the facts, they can be a compass to lead me in the right direction. There are certain things I now know I can do to create comfort for myself. This may include running myself a warm bath, making myself a cup of tea, or taking a drive up the California coast—while allowing myself to sob and express the full range of my emotions. Other comforts: listening to certain musical tracks, preparing myself nurturing food, visiting an outdoor farmer's market. Sometimes I feel best when I am alone, and at other times I reach out to the people who allow me to feel heard and understood.

In the past, I could not trust my choices in confidantes and my ability to listen to my heart. I feared that, if I allowed myself to *feel*, it would become a bottomless pit of despair. That once I started, I would not be able to stop. The opposite was true. My emotions and tears were like a bath cleansing me from the inside out. Self-soothing and self-mothering are healing.

There is another version of mothering that I am experiencing now: babying myself. To me this means paying special attention to my needs. In the past, I could reach out for a chocolate bar or a pint of ice cream when I was in a difficult place, but now, if I am on the case as my own best advocate, I know what those treats will do to me after the short-term benefits of instant gratification are gone. The mother in me provides discipline and boundaries. So now, I fulfill the needs of the real baby in me by sipping water throughout the day. This is a constant soothing and nurturing action and a reminder that the mother in me is present. I also prepare my meals, chopping the vegetables in advance, making sure that I get my servings of dark leafy greens. I avoid dehydrating goodies. I create space, allowing myself all the time I need to factor in this nurturing. These small and constant acts become the foundation for the healing process. Allowing the feelings to come, while also providing the stabilizing antidote, is the mothering that I have been looking for. It's what we all need.

Love your emotions! Feelings are a gift, so let them flow freely. Watch where emotions lead you and know that this flow is creative. Mothering is the most creative action, as a mother can create an entire human being. That creative force is within you and rides on the currents of your emotions. Have the courage to dive in and feel it all.

SELF-LOVE CHECKLIST
YOGALOSOPHY FOR INNER STRENGTH program

- ❑ **Sunday:** Be Happy Yoga
- ❑ **Monday:** Back-to-Basics Yoga
- ❑ **Tuesday:** Cardio
- ❑ **Wednesday:** Bounce Back! Yoga
- ❑ **Thursday:** Day Off
- ❑ **Friday:** Let Go Yoga
- ❑ **Saturday:** Get Strong Yogalosophy
- ❑ **Heart-Opening Pose:** Camel
- ❑ **Love Movement:** Go Swimming
- ❑ **Heart-Healing Meditation:** Heart Forgiveness With a Parent Meditation
- ❑ **Love Notes:** How Do You Feel Today?
- ❑ **Ritual:** Hugs and Hands
- ❑ **Strength for the Soul:** Yell, Sob, Laugh

MANTRA

I am full of feeling and compassion. I courageously take responsibility for my needs and the full range of my human emotion. I nurture, protect, empower, and initiate myself.

TRACK OF THE WEEK

"10,000 Emerald Pools" by BØRNS or "This Is to Mother You" by Sinéad O'Connor

HEART-OPENING POSE: CAMEL

Camel Pose is an apex pose, which means it is a more challenging posture that requires proper warm-ups—standing postures specific to the area of the body that the posture targets—until you build up to it. After you've built up to the apex pose, you begin to cool your body down. Apex poses should be done once your body is warm. You may add this to one of your routines after you have opened your shoulders, loosened your spine, and stretched your hips. Once you have done so you may attempt this pose.

- Begin in a kneeling position with your knees hip-width apart.

- Press your shins into the mat and internally rotate your thighs toward the inner thigh area; this will release your back. (NOTE: avoid clenching your butt.)

- Place your hands on your lower back for support, and look forward as you lean back, pressing the hips forward.

- To deepen the pose, you may take one of the hands onto the same heel and arc the opposite arm overhead, reaching back as you gaze at the fingertips. If you do this, hold for several breaths

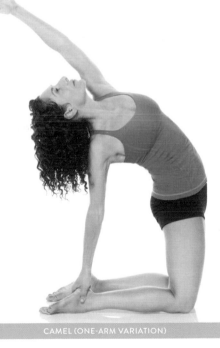

CAMEL (ONE-ARM VARIATION)

- If you feel this in your lower back at all, modify by tucking your toes. This should make it easier to grab your heels. Keep your hips pressing forward so that they are directly above your knees.

- Keep your lower spine long. You may let your head drop back or keep it neutral. Relax and open the shoulders. Hold for 30 to 60 seconds.

- To rise out of this, bring the palms together in prayer, then lead with your heart and lift your torso as you press your hips forward. Your head should be the last to rise.

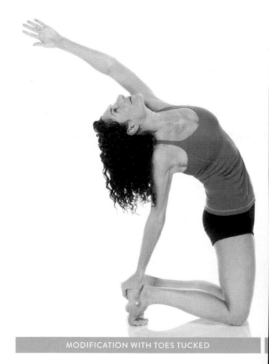

MODIFICATION WITH TOES TUCKED

LOVE MOVEMENT: GO SWIMMING

Go swimming: in the ocean, in a lake, or in a pool. If you swim in a pool, swim in the deep end. If you're able to dive, I dare you to dive. This will invoke the feeling of courage that it takes to do so, so you'll have a physical experience of courage. Courage does not mean you do not feel fear. It is feeling that fear *and* going forward anyway that is brave. If we never felt even a little scared, we would never experience courage.

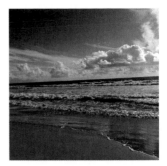

LAUREN'S STORY

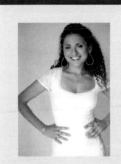

Certified holistic nutritionist and lifestyle coach Lauren Haas helps private and corporate clients reach their optimum health in realistic ways. She is also one of my former students and a sister in self-love through healthy living. Her story is inspiration to follow your emotions no matter what things look like on the outside, and to mother yourself in the kitchen. Find her recipes on pages 219 and 221.

• • •

Lauren

Food simultaneously tantalizes all five of your senses and is also a direct channel for nourishing your body, mind, and spirit. So if you have an illness, and you discover that what you're eating is the root cause, a sense of loss takes over.

Most of my life, I struggled with digestive problems, weight gain, skin issues, and a twisted relationship with food. When I found out that nutritional allergies were the cause of my health issues, I had to stop eating a long list of foods.

I couldn't enjoy a rich, creamy bowl of ice cream or a fluffy, buttery croissant, in fear that I would get sick. Food was no longer pleasurable and became a burden. I fell into a downward spiral. I felt a loss of control over my life and the only thing that I could control was the food on my plate. My love for food became a fear, which manifested into an eating disorder.

Eventually, I hit rock bottom.

Coincidently, during this time I was working as a private holistic chef and my life was filled with food, but I missed the joy of eating. I had to take a deep look at myself. I decided that I had to make a change.

I went straight into the kitchen and dedicated myself to creating original dishes, like gluten-free chocolate chip cookies, that I could eat. While food took my "life" away, eventually food also gave me my life back—because through this experience I found my purpose in life: I heal people with food. I bring the joy of health and eating back into the lives of people who are saddened by the same loss I went through.

HEART-HEALING MEDITATION: HEART FORGIVENESS WITH A PARENT MEDITATION

Many of our emotional wounds can be resolved with forgiveness. Forgive and be forgiven. You may want forgiveness because you have felt anger or even hatred toward your own parents. You may need to forgive them for the actions they took against you.

Underneath it all, there is universal love that is bigger than all of it. When my father walked out on my mother for another woman, he wrote me a note that I wasn't ready to digest. It said, "Forgiveness is more for the forgiver than for the one who is forgiven." Although I didn't want to admit it at the time, it turns out he was right. This week's meditation is a forgiveness practice.

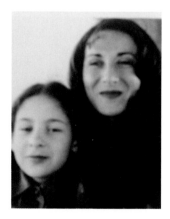

Find a quiet and safe space. Get into a comfortable position and close your eyes. Take three long, slow, deep breaths. Send the breath throughout your body, feeling the life force energy moving through you. Bring your awareness to your heart space and sense how you feel in this moment. Imagine seeing your parent (either mother or father) in front of you, and imagine their heart sitting right on top of your heart. Sit and breathe with your parent's ethereal heart and your ethereal heart together. After 5 or 10 or 20 minutes say silently or out loud: "I love you. I forgive you. Please forgive me. Thank you." Repeat these words several times until you feel complete. Sit with the feeling of your mother or your father on your heart and breathe. When you feel complete, give yourself a hug.

LOVE NOTES: HOW DO YOU FEEL TODAY?

See if you are able to identify how you feel daily. Choose from the list of emotions shown in the Strength for the Soul section to follow and write a few paragraphs about how you feel every day this week. You are beginning a dialogue with your true self.

RITUAL: HUGS AND HANDS

This week I have two rituals for you.

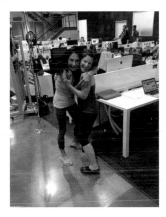

Ritual one: During the day, get five hugs. I tried this experiment myself because I kept hearing that hugs have an actual physiological effect on the body. See this chapter's Heart Fact (page 217) for the benefits! What's wonderful about hugging is that you get to give and receive at the same time. That is mothering at its finest. It also takes courage to reach out for a hug.

Ritual two: At night, when you're in bed, hold your own hand. I have actually had a wonderful feeling of intimacy when I hold my own hand. I know I am not alone because one of my dear yoga teacher friends told me he actually puts his own arms around himself when he sleeps—because he found out in therapy that, emotionally, you don't really know the difference. There is a soothing quality to touch, even if it is your own. I have recently found a new favorite comforting touch: a hot water bottle. I really love the warmth of another being in the bed with me, so the hot water bottle has been a godsend! I highly recommend it. So this week, fill a water bottle with hot water from the tap, get a towel to buffer the heat if necessary, and cuddle up.

I learned the following lesson in acting class. It allows you to express all of your basic human emotions: anger, sadness, joy. Even if you are faking it, it's a good way to exercise your emotional muscles. Set a timer and express each for one minute: 1) yelling, 2) sobbing, 3) laughing. You can start off just faking it. You may very well end up feeling the real thing. It's very healthy to feel. This is taking responsibility for feeling.

Here is a list of emotions to help you identify how you feel. This is also the list you can draw from when doing your Love Notes this week. Feel free to add to this list as you get to know yourself better.

HAPPINESS: Loved. Joyful. Awed. Hopeful. Caring. Elated. Exhilarated. Playful. Ecstatic. Peaceful. Excited. Content. Adventurous. Daring. Intrigued. Fascinated. Pleased. Overjoyed. Thrilled. Passionate. Cheerful. Gratified. Satisfied. Glowing. Mellow. Pleased. Confident. Brave. Friendly. Proud. Strong. Thankful.

JEALOUSY: Betrayed. Envious. Possessive. Unloved. Unsafe. Irrational. Rejected. Suspicious. Intolerant.

PAIN: Defeated. Disappointed. Unworthy. Ashamed. Despondent. Cheated. Suffering. Unhappy. Forlorn. Despair. Depressed. Discontented. Regret.

REJECTION: Abandoned. Awkward. Powerless. Misunderstood. Foolish. Lonely. Insecure. Apathetic. Helpless. Exasperated.

ANGER: Enraged. Furious. Outraged. Irate. Upset. Mad. Disgusted. Agitated. Seething. Defensive. Annoyed. Perturbed. Resistant. Irritated. Touchy. Aggressive. Resentful. Hostile.

AFRAID: Anxious. Unsure. Timid. Worried. Nervous. Cautious. Terrified. Horrified. Frantic. Shocked. Petrified. Apprehensive. Threatened. Frightened. Uneasy. Intimidated. Concerned. Guarded. Vulnerable. Tense. Frozen.

ASHAMED: Bashful. Unworthy. Guilty. Embarrassed. Mortified. Dishonored. Worthless. Defamed. Remorseful. Sorrowful.

SAD: Depressed. Alone. Dejected. Sorrowful. Heartbroken. Somber. Lost. Melancholy. Let down. Blue. Moody. Dissatisfied. Apathetic. Raw. Weak. Stuck. Disillusioned.

 Hugging lowers the levels of the stress hormone cortisol, and increases the level of the "love hormone" oxytocin. According to one study, a 10-second hug lowers the risk of heart disease because it boosts your immune system, eases depression, fights fatigue, and reduces stress—increasing your happiness and emotional vitality.

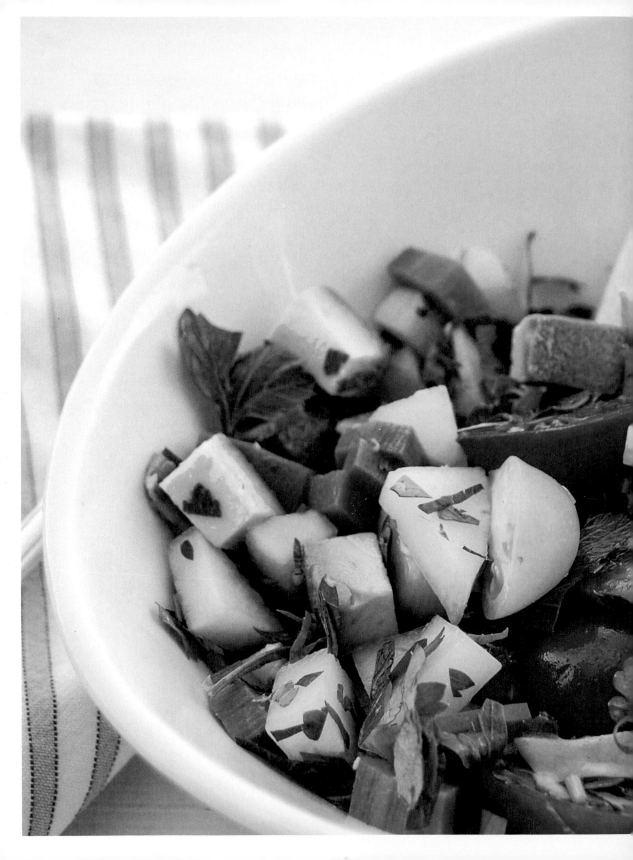

HAAS HOLISTIC HEART-HEALING CHOPPED SALAD

Serves 4—6

This salad, which can serve as a side dish or be eaten alone as a meal, is chock-full of whole, healthy ingredients! The avocado alone provides monounsaturated fat (the healthy kind of fat), as well as nearly twenty vitamins and minerals. Artichokes are a good source of dietary fiber, and the pickled ginger is great for digestion. Consume with this in mind: as above, so below. What do I mean by this? Reminding yourself of the benefits of your food can aid in the way your body receives the medicine.

1 PACK OR 1 CAN ARTICHOKE HEARTS

1 ENGLISH CUCUMBER

2 CARROTS

1 CUP CHERRY TOMATOES

1 BUNCH CILANTRO OR PARSLEY

1 AVOCADO

JUICE OF 1 LEMON (2 TO 3 TABLESPOONS)

1 TABLESPOON ALMOND OIL

2 TABLESPOONS SEASONED RICE WINE VINEGAR*

2 TABLESPOONS DIJON MUSTARD

1 TABLESPOON COCONUT LIQUID AMINOS

2 TABLESPOONS MINCED PICKLED GINGER (SUSHI GINGER)

SALT AND PEPPER

Note: Make sure to use seasoned rice wine vinegar. If the vinegar isn't seasoned, the dressing will be very tart.

Dice all the vegetables except the avocado into $1/2$-inch cubes. Cut tomatoes in half and chop the cilantro/parsley. Place everything in a large bowl and set it aside.

Cube the avocado and set it aside in a small bowl. Squeeze/sprinkle lemon juice over the avocado to keep it from turning brown.

To make the salad dressing, place the almond oil, seasoned rice wine vinegar, Dijon mustard, coconut liquid aminos, and ginger in a mason jar with a tight-fitting lid. Shake the jar until all ingredients are combined.

When ready to serve, toss the salad with the dressing and top with the cubed avocado.

Recipe by Lauren Haas

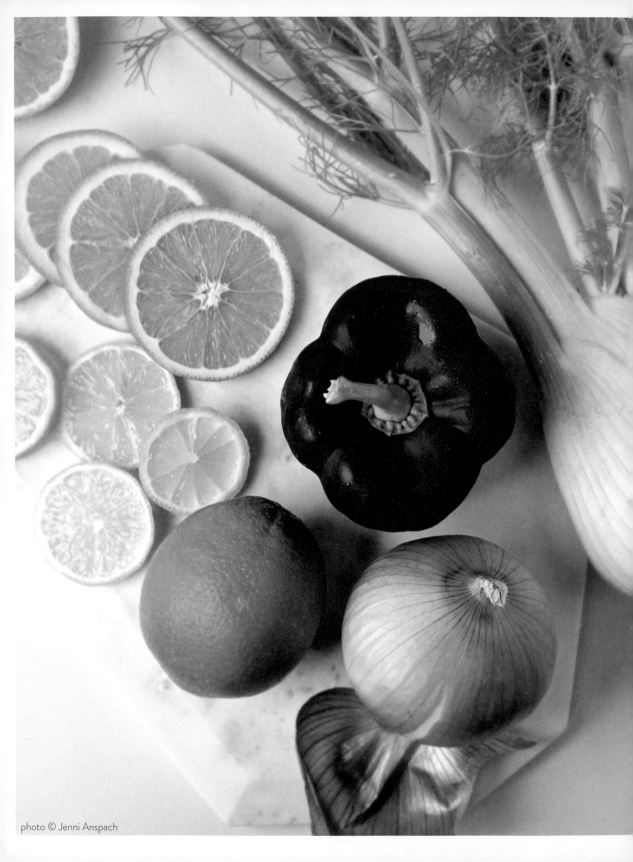

ROASTED CITRUS TROUT WITH FENNEL, PEPPERS, ONION, AND GINGER

Serves 2

This dish takes a little bit of work, but that's the point! As a labor of love, cooking can be a great therapeutic way to nurture yourself. Keep that intention in mind as you lovingly prepare this dish.

2 LEMONS: 1 FOR JUICE, 1 CUT IN SLICES (WITH PEEL)

1 NAVEL ORANGE OR 2 SMALL ORANGES

2 TABLESPOONS MINCED PICKLED GINGER (SUSHI GINGER)

2 TABLESPOONS DIJON MUSTARD

1 TABLESPOON COCONUT LIQUID AMINOS

SALT AND PEPPER

GRAPE SEED OIL

1 SWEET YELLOW ONION, SLICED IN ¼-INCH HALF MOONS

1 BELL PEPPER, SLICED IN ¼-INCH STRIPS

1 FENNEL BULB, SLICED IN ¼-INCH MOONS

COCONUT OIL

2 SMALL WHOLE TROUT, DEBONED (ASK THE FISHMONGER TO DO THIS FOR YOU)

Preheat oven to 450°F.

To make the marinade, combine the juice from 1 lemon, ½ navel orange/1 small orange, minced pickled ginger, mustard, coconut liquid aminos, and salt in a bowl. Set aside.

Heat a pan with grape seed oil. Add the onion, pepper, fennel, 1 sliced lemon (with peel), and remaining orange (also sliced, with its peel). Sauté until soft and golden. Season with salt and pepper.

Grease with coconut oil a roasting pan large enough to fit both fish. Place two-thirds of the cooked vegetables (peppers, fennel, lemon, and orange) in the roasting pan. Set the rest of the vegetables aside.

Season the trout inside and out with salt and pepper. Pour the ginger-mustard marinade inside both fillets, spreading evenly. Stuff both fillets with the remaining fennel, peppers, onions, lemon, and orange slices. Close the fillets.

Place stuffed fish over the vegetables. Put in the oven and cook for 15 to 30 minutes, depending on the size of your fish. (Smaller fish will cook in 15 to 20 minutes; larger fish will cook in 20 to 30 minutes.)

Remove from oven and check to see if fish are cooked through. Perfectly cooked trout will be nearly opaque, moist, and will flake easily with a fork. If your fish isn't cooked, place back in the oven and cook for 5 minutes or until fish is opaque.

Serve fish and vegetables together. Enjoy!

Recipe by Lauren Haas

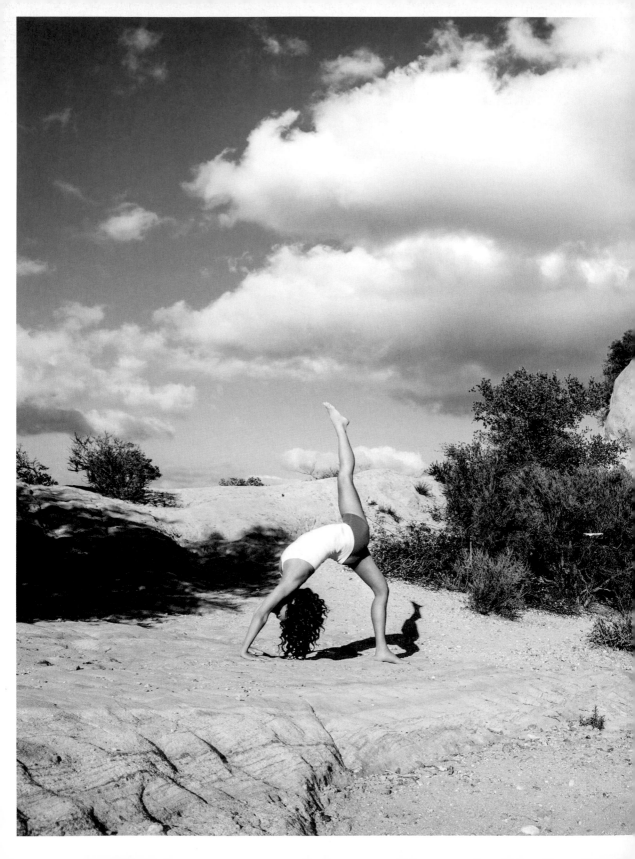

WEEK 5

Jump-start Your Heart

The heart is the gateway between the physical realm and the higher realms. The heart is able to integrate the body, mind, and spirit and can translate it into the universal language of *feeling*—of love. In yoga, we practice being in the heart space and the love for spirit because it gives us a sense of belonging and a connection to our higher purpose.

The heart, being both physical and subtle, must be exercised in a variety of ways: energetically, emotionally, soulfully, and physically. I consider physical exercise a tangible offering of thanks for my body. Cardiovascular work lifts your spirits and literally strengthens (and enlarges) your heart. You stretch your capacity for intensity. You create room for discomfort, as a compassionate witness, and then move past that feeling of wanting to give up, striving toward the next level of excellence. In this way, physical activity that pushes you to an anaerobic state can be a living model for moving through the pain of brokenness. Both aerobic and anaerobic exercises are essential to heart health. Aerobic exercise, which most of us know, is for fat burning and cardiovascular conditioning. What you may not know is that it is essential to occasionally work anaerobically and exceed your comfort zone in order to increase your performance and strive for excellence. This elevates your fitness level so that you are able to increase your capacity to do even more. It's a literal training for witnessing

> "The heart is positive. Just as mind says no, the heart says yes."
>
> —OSHO, FROM *EMOTIONAL WELLNESS: TRANSFORMING FEAR, ANGER, AND JEALOUSY INTO CREATIVE ENERGY*

your struggle, with love, which even allows for a sweetness, and pleasure in the sensation. Similar to reframing with the words you say, once you notice how pleasurable the physical sensation of your struggle can be, you send an entirely new message to yourself about your capacity for kindness, growth, and strength.

After emotional distress, your heart enlarges as well, opening up to all sorts of new experiences, places, and ways to receive and give love. Of course hurt is one of the best access points to your true center. The pain that grabs you when you are experiencing a loss will lead you to a new level of self-awareness. There are always advantages and blessings to count. During trying times, friendships can become more fulfilling and important; even connections with total strangers are blessings. We grow in compassion for others in pain. There is a rekindling of the passion for meaning. We can say "yes" to life and be grateful for the simplest things as a way of becoming more empowered on our way out of the wreckage of the past.

This week we will jump-start your heart, get in touch with your inner child, move your legs to move you forward, and even make art out of all that delicious heartfelt emotion that you set free. Plus, you'll even have fun doing it!

✹ MY STORY

I recall the time I spent with one of my closest friends when she was going through a painful and public divorce. Everybody was *Mad About* Helen Hunt in the late nineties and beyond. She was everyone's dream wife. On screen she was sharp, hilarious, the sexy girl next door, and a best friend to her on-screen husband, costar Paul Reiser. Helen also happened to be pretty much the same in real life. She is one of my own dearest friends, and attended my Santa Monica Spinning classes daily. Yes, we had a lot of soul in our cycle, even in my nineties classes. Helen had been with actor Hank Azaria (well known for his voices on *The Simpsons* and a host of other wide-ranging parts) for a while. Hank was my dear friend as well, and equally funny, charismatic, and down-to-earth. Following a sweet wedding, the union unraveled, as these things can. Although I have never been married, I am a romantic and I want marriages to work. This one fizzled, and it was very public for a very private person.

Due to my own family history, being a bystander is my specialty, and I am very good to be around during transitional times. I honestly believe that witnessing my parents' breakup and the deterioration of their relationship was my training for witnessing those dear to me experiencing similar moments. At the time, I had not yet had firsthand experience of breakup. I was still in my fairy tale romance, and the public spotlight had yet to fall upon me. But I was most certainly willing to be present for my friends' process. And I was.

Spinning was a large part of her healing process. In fact, many of my students used Spinning as a heart healing tool. Physical expression and high energy not only helps by giving that endorphin rush, but it also takes the edge off the aggression and pent-up energy. Plus, it's fun! I always say: if you want to move forward, move your legs. Helen and I began with this major component. Then there was fun to be had—getting henna tattoos on the Venice boardwalk, going to movies, or having lunch at the beach—these were other types of activities we would do. We found ways to ritualize the breakup. It's great to have a trusted friend who already knows the details of your particular heartbreak, so that you can focus on letting go of the story and just find ways to have fun and play.

Helen and I have witnessed one another through many moments of grief, including the global loss of September 11, 2001, also known as 9/11.

On the heels of a budding new romance, Helen, her new beau, Matthew, and I took a trip to New York City to go to the U.S. Open. She was trying to turn me into a tennis fan, always getting me to play and have fun. We were scheduled to fly home on an 11:00 AM flight to Los Angeles from JFK on September 11, 2001. We woke up early to grab breakfast at the joint below her swanky Manhattan loft, located nine blocks away from the World Trade Center. I noted it was a gorgeous sunny morning as we walked to Bubbie's Deli.

"Let's sit by the window, so we can look out at the view," I suggested excitedly. We sat down for our breakfast on this astonishingly beautiful morning when I heard something crash, like thunder. I looked out to see papers and what appeared to be glitter, but what I now assume was glass, falling from the World Trade Center. "It looks like a celebration," I said innocently.

A group of people gathered outside were looking at a hole in the building. We joined. I was a bit afraid that there had been an explosion, but when someone pointed out the hole, and the tail of the plane sticking out, I felt relief that it was a freak accident. I could see people waving from the tower that had been hit. The restaurant owner turned on the television, to that image of the two buildings, but there was no explanation.

Helen and I decided to go in and scarf our breakfast while her boyfriend went to get our bags to put in the car and get out of the city ASAP. As I was sitting in a daze with my eggs and berries, experiencing the weirdness with Helen, I saw the explosion of the second plane hitting the other tower and in an instant knew that this was bad. The restaurant owner dropped to his knees. Everything seemed fast and slow all at once. We rushed out and to her loft. As we gathered our things I suggested turning on the television. Once the Pentagon was hit everything unfolded rapidly and we knew we were stuck in NYC.

When the World Trade Center buildings came down, I sat at the edge of the bed where we had been huddled in front of the television. Not only could we watch it on TV but we could literally feel the rumbling and the shaking as the buildings came down. I remember preparing myself for death. Yes, I prayed for safety, even in my death. I imagined a vessel of light. I closed my eyes, connected to my breath, and prayed . . . That sort of thing. We really lucked out that the wind was blowing in the direction it was blowing because we were preparing to be covered in debris, unable to see out of the windows. Instead, the billows of smoke from the fire blew away from us.

The neighborhood was covered in dust and Lord knows what toxic particles from the building, all in an overlay of death. We remained in the loft space for another five hours, but then were evacuated when Building 7 went down later that afternoon and from there were on the run. Matthew got me a mask from one of the cops, and we booked uptown in fear. The next several days are an odyssey that felt like a combination of refuge and an adult haunted house that had us frozen and arrested in terror. I wanted desperately to get home, particularly because my father was set to have chemotherapy for his lymphoma, and it had not gone so well the previous time. Let's just call this a heightened moment in my life.

Days later, we made it home on one of the first jets out of Allentown, Pennsylvania. Don't ask me how it happened, but it was a miracle and also the shortest flight of my life. Once we landed, my boyfriend picked me up and I got up early the next morning to teach my 7:00 AM Spinning class. I will never forget my dear friend and student Dave Garber greeting me in the street and me saying how there were helicopters overhead—only to register his look at me as if to say: *No. There are no helicopters.* I was in full-blown PTSD.

The class I taught was wordless. The only two musical artists I could think of playing were U2, who were born from war and dissention, and Peter Gabriel, who emanates depth of emotion. I made it a point to go to each person in that room, all fifty of them, and to have a moment of connection where I allowed them to look into my eyes and see my pain, and I shared their pain by seeing them. It was all I could do, and it was very healing. It was all I had.

It's wonderful to be able to express how you feel, but continually retelling the story of your anguish doesn't always make you feel lighter. When talking about it over and over again no longer helps you to let go, then what?

So here's the catch: when you are not in your head, and you are not trying to figure it out, where does that leave you? Feeling! Oh, how uncomfortable it is to be transparent and vulnerable. When I'm in my heart I might have to feel uncomfortable, squishy feelings of insecurity, loneliness, abandonment, and shame. All of the feelings from childhood woes come flooding forth, and then what? Well, the heart is big enough for all of it. The heart makes art, poetry, music, and films with its vulnerability. The heart gets bigger than all of the complexities, and contains the oceans of opposites without separation. The heart is accustomed to this fine-tuning of life's events and transforms tragic beauty into soulful songs, fine art, and epic movies. The heart is fiery and it burns the ego, knowing that this is simply a moment in time, and that more is to be shown to you. "Everything works out in the end, and if it hasn't worked out, it's not the end." I've seen it time and again. There was a Matthew that was the antidote to Hank. Just when you thought Brad Pitt was the catch of all time, along came the arguably sexier Justin Theroux. In the end even 9/11 became a reference point for me. It didn't ruin me. It was a loss of innocence, yet it woke me up. What had I been thinking all those years—feeling less a part of the world because I hadn't experienced raw human loss on a global level. All I am saying is: you just don't know what's up ahead or around the corner. Anything is possible and anything can become an opportunity, especially if you make room for it.

SELF-LOVE CHECKLIST

YOGALOSOPHY FOR INNER STRENGTH program

- ☐ **Sunday:** Be Happy Yoga
- ☐ **Monday:** Back-to-Basics Yoga
- ☐ **Tuesday:** Cardio
- ☐ **Wednesday:** Bounce Back! Yoga
- ☐ **Thursday:** Day Off
- ☐ **Friday:** Let Go Yoga
- ☐ **Saturday:** Get Strong Yogalosophy
- ☐ **Heart-Opening Pose:** Wheel With Leg Extended
- ☐ **Love Movement:** Playful Childhood Activity
- ☐ **Heart-Healing Meditation:** Heart Pulse With Mudra
- ☐ **Love Notes:** Write to Your Child Self
- ☐ **Ritual:** Attend a Kitran
- ☐ **Strength for the Soul:** Say "Yes!"
- ☐ **Art Break for Heartbreak:**
  - The Love Letter
  - Art Therapy

MANTRA

My heart is opening. I am loved, loving, and lovable. My tears are an investment in my future happiness.

TRACK OF THE WEEK

"In Your Eyes" (live version) by Peter Gabriel, or "Bad" by U2.

HEART-OPENING POSE: WHEEL WITH LEG EXTENDED

Wheel is an aspirational, or apex pose, which is a more strenuous posture and must be practiced after a sufficient warm-up. Preparing with shoulder openers and standing postures will warm the upper body and build the leg strength needed for Wheel.

Wheel is also a backbend. Backbends are always heart openers and tend to lift our spirits. They also stretch out the entire front of the body. Sometimes when the front of the body is tight you can experience that as back pain; Wheel provides your front with a good stretch. It's a great posture to target the kidneys and adrenal glands—which will energize you more than a cup of coffee (I swear!).

Everybody is unique, and you must connect with yourself first. I recommend consulting with someone in person who can assist you in building up to this posture safely. So, mostly, play and have fun. If it's not fun, don't do it! Here are the instructions:

- From a supine position, place your feet on the floor with your knees bent. Feel the support of the floor beneath you, which supports your spine so it is in alignment. Bend your elbows and place your hands with palms on the floor, by your ears, and fingers directing toward your shoulders.

- Press the shoulders down into the floor, lengthen your back by drawing the tailbone in, and press your feet into the floor.

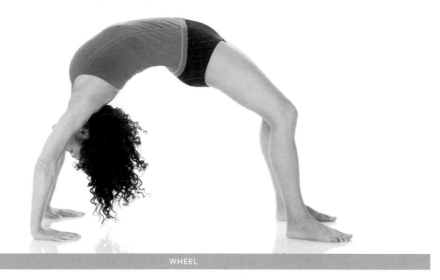

WHEEL

- Take a deep breath in. As you exhale, peel your back off the mat and press your hips up to the ceiling. Hang out for several breaths.

- Breathe in. As you breathe out, pull your feet in toward yourself and draw your shoulder blades onto your back. Pull your armpits in and press your hands down to lift your body up. (Take this in stages.) Place the crown of the head on the floor, and pause. Then press down to lift, and straighten your arms as much as you can.

- Aim your toes straight ahead, and keep your knees aligned over your toes. If this is straining your lower back, you may try elevating onto the toes. Internally rotate your thighs. Lengthen your tailbone. Allow your head to hang down.

- If you want to take this to the next level, allow your head to hang; keeping your upper arm externally rotating, draw your right knee in. Then extend the leg so your toes reach for the ceiling. Hold for a breath or two, and then switch sides.

- After several breaths here, prepare to come down. Tucking your chin slightly and softly, slowly lower yourself, vertebra by vertebra, down to the floor.

- To release the spine, draw the knees into your chest and rock gently from side to side.

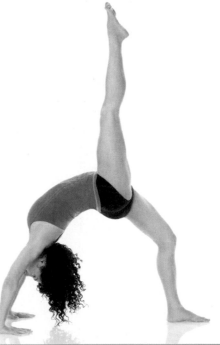

WHEEL WITH LEG EXTENDED

LOVE MOVEMENT:
PLAYFUL CHILDHOOD ACTIVITY

Jumping rope is one of the most challenging cardiovascular exercises available—and it reminds us
of when we were kids! So I highly recommend
this. But if you're not drawn to it, try something
else fun. Maybe a hip-hop dance class, or samba.
I've seen some awesome women hoop dancing
with a modern day hula hoop, which is both playful and sexy. What calls to you and makes you feel
young? Do that.

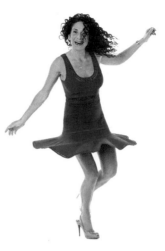

JAVIERA'S STORY

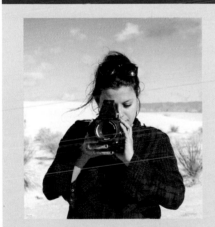

This week's contributor is my dear friend Javiera
Estrada, fine artist and photographer of this book.
She offers her two Art Break for Heart Break rituals in the Strength for the Soul section on pages
236 and 237. Here is her story:

• • •

Javiera

I was seventeen years old when I fell in love for
the first time. Young and full of expectations, I
believed in the myth of finding my soul mate and
running off into the sunset. Years later, the relationship revealed itself to be emotionally damaging and it became crystal clear that my "soul mate" was not what I expected.
This reality was devastating. The experience hurled me into one of the most challenging
times of my life. Angry, attached, and depressed, I found myself utterly heartbroken
and unable to fathom my life without this person. The intensity of sadness that en-
gulfed my being was overwhelming. And yet, simultaneously I could also glimpse a little
sparkle hidden deep within that cave of darkness, waiting to be chiseled out.

At the time I was not living as an artist but, always creative, I decided to channel all of my feelings into splashing some color on whatever I could get my hands on. My home became a jumble of canvas, paints, papers, collages, pens, photographs, inks, and brushes. All I could do was paint, all day every day, in order to cope with my emotions. I soon realized this experience was a major blessing, for it catapulted me into becoming the artist I am today. I am grateful to my "soul mate" for revealing these hidden treasures that today bring me so much joy. My view on relationships has dramatically changed since that first love, and I find them to be great opportunities for growth and self-reflection. True love is the art of forgiveness and loving unconditionally. Every day we are gifted the opportunity to practice this, and each person is a jewel for us to polish our skills. Therefore, embrace heartbreak—for you never know what blessings you may receive.

HEART-HEALING MEDITATION: HEART PULSE WITH MUDRA

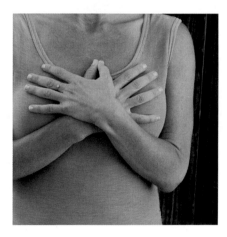

The idea is to connect with your own heartbeat, with your own pulse. It's a beautiful feeling, and all it requires is that you pay attention to your heart. Lie down and place one hand, palm down and fingers spread, at the center of your chest. Place the other palm gently on top of it, connecting the thumbs to touch. It should almost look like an angel or bird with wings over your heart. This is a heart-opening mudra. Close your eyes and simply observe your pulse as you breathe normally. Remain here, observing and sensing your pulse for 10 minutes, and notice how calm you are after that time.

LOVE NOTES: WRITE TO YOUR CHILD SELF

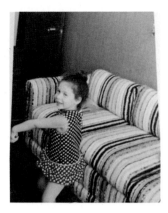

Write a letter to your child self from your adult self. Tell her what happens as the story of your future unfolds, and that everything is going to be okay. Imagine that you could elevate yourself above the time line of your life. You would have the unique perspective of a pattern. The map of your life could resemble a tapestry of all that had ever happened to you thus far and all that was possible in the future. From this place of wisdom, you can reach forward or backward as you choose. You can see your entire life. You can see that as life takes its twists and turns, it always brings you to a place of resolution. Life has a way of integrating all of the experiences that make you the incredible being that you are now. So write a really good letter to that little one, telling her how much she has to look forward to.

RITUAL: ATTEND A KIRTAN

Kirtan is chanting, or call-and-response. This is much more than singing—it's an act of *bhakti*, also called the yoga of devotional love. The most beautiful times I have had within the yoga community are these chants. (I can recommend both a live Steve Ross *kirtan* at Maha Yoga in Los Angeles—Steve Ross has a CD called "Give Love a Chants"—and Krishna Das, a Grammy-nominated kirtan artist who tours the world. You can go to Krishna Das's website to see his tour dates, download one of his CDs, or find someone in your community with a humble kirtan practice.)

Chanting is devotional and joyful. When you sing, the blissful energy of sound vibrates through your body and can help to heal your heart. Not only that, but when you're singing in a group, it really doesn't matter if you have a "good" voice. With call-and-response, you won't have to memorize anything. It's simply repetition. Repetition will bring you bliss. In and of itself, it is a meditation. Even if you don't understand the words you are saying, you can feel the connection of celebration in expressing gratitude and love to the universe. If you are strongly opposed to trying a chant, or that is not available to you in your hometown, you can sing your heart out at karaoke. When one of my favorite and most fun clients, Kate Beckinsale, was in a particularly down mood, she went out and sang at a karaoke bar and brought her spirits soaring into yoga the next day. If it works for her, it can work for you.

STRENGTH FOR THE SOUL: SAY "YES!"

Say "yes" this week. Notice the things that come your way, and say, "Yes!" We often get into a habitual pattern of cutting ourselves off from the opportunities the universe offers. Consider the universe your playmate, and the opportunities that are presented to you as part of your playground. Watch your world open as you notice the habitual "no" and choose "yes" instead.

ask the expert

TAKE AN ART BREAK FOR YOUR HEART BREAK: TWO RITUALS BY JAVIERA ESTRADA

THE LOVE LETTER

I find whenever I'm feeling "stuck" on negative emotions or want to let go of something, I always write a letter to the person in question. The first letter is unfiltered, raw, and charged with emotion and unrestrained craziness. Once I get all of that out, I burn it and start writing my second letter. Sometimes after I burn the first one, I feel satisfied and don't feel the need to write another. But there are also times where I have written over twenty letters! Yup. There's no limit to how many letters you may write. The purpose isn't to send them necessarily, but to purge any unspoken feelings in order to clear them. I have been doing this since I was a teenager, and I must say it's a great tool when you need to process! All you need is pen and paper. It's that easy!

ART THERAPY

Another way of healing from challenging times can be processing emotions through art. You don't have to be a professional "artist" or have gone to school for art in order to be creative. I never went to art school, can't draw a stick figure, and here I am making art. That being said, we are all artists in one shape or another. You can use whatever you have lying around the house—such as paper, pencils, markers or paints—and just start creating. Don't overanalyze or critique your skills because it's not about that. If I thought about how awful my drawing skills were, I would have never started! Also, you're not making a Picasso here—this is for you and for you only. There is a big difference between making art to sell and art therapy. I don't tend to show anyone my therapy art because it's very personal and, honestly, I don't think anyone would like to hang a portrait of my ex-boyfriend's severed head. Ha. :)

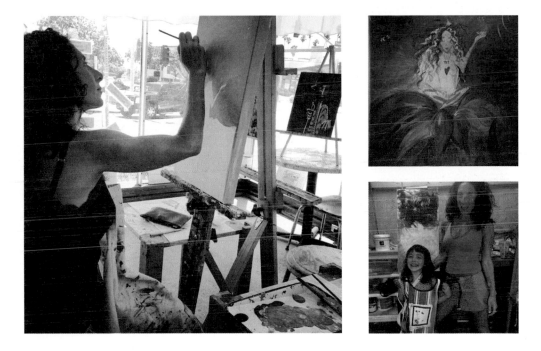

HEART FACT On average, your heart beats 100,000 times a day. The Earth has a heartbeat, too: a frequency of 8 Hz. When you pair that with your brain waves, listening to 432 Hz music allows you to tune into and resonate with a feeling of well-being and peace.

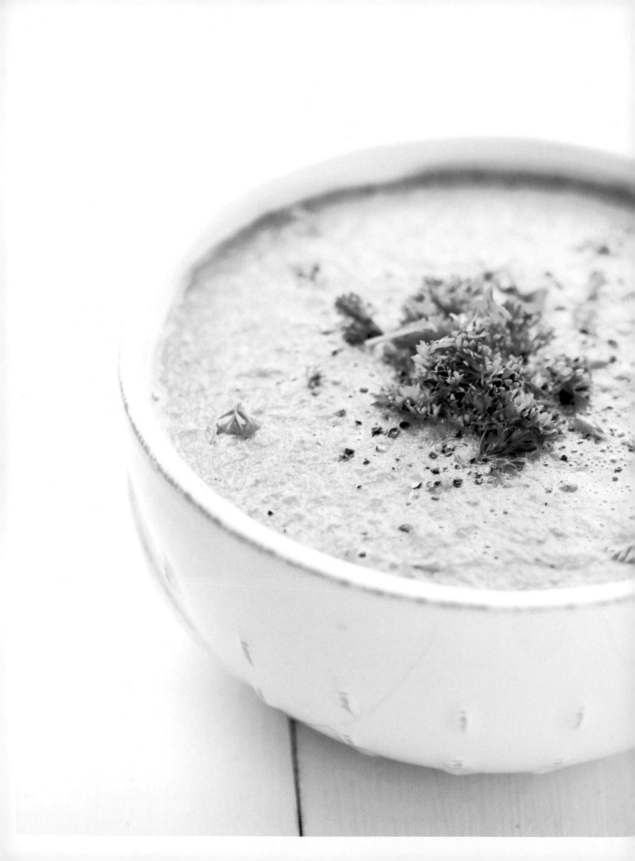

GLORIOUS GREEN MACHINE SOUP

Serves 2—4

Connect with your heart and think about how healthy greens are for your blood and how the heart is going to pump that healthy blood to all of your extremities. Talk to your food with a prayer of thanks. Then consume.

1 CUP CHOPPED CURLY KALE

1 CUP CHOPPED ZUCCHINI (OR PACKAGED JULIENNE-CUT BROCCOLI)

1 CUP CHOPPED DANDELION GREENS (OR DARK LEAFY GREEN OF YOUR CHOICE, SUCH AS CHARD OR WATERCRESS)

1 RIPE AVOCADO, HALVED

½ LEMON

SALT TO TASTE

PEPPER TO TASTE

2 CUPS WATER

COCONUT OIL, FOR DRIZZLING

Boil 2 cups of water.

Put the curly kale, zucchini, and your choice of greens in a heat-safe blender. Squeeze in half a lemon. Pour 1–2 cups boiling water over the vegetables. Add salt and pepper to taste.

Blend for 30 seconds and then add half the avocado. Blend to desired thickness. Pour into the bowl. Slice the remaining avocado and add to the bowl to give it texture. Drizzle coconut oil over the soup and serve.

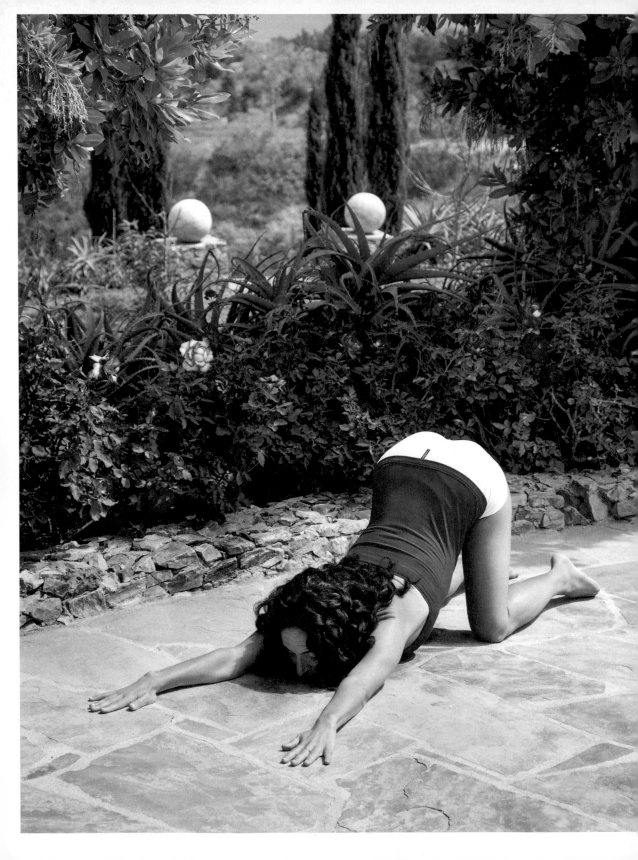

WEEK 6

Reach Out from Your Compassion

When you feel "love," what you are feeling is your own loving nature coming through. It's not coming from someone else. It's radiating from inside you, and is, theoretically, yours to conjure up at any time. But during periods of great sadness or loss, it's hard to find pathways to access it. This week I'm going to help you tap into that love and show you that, even when you feel empty, you are enough, you have enough love to share to help another, and that in reaching out and giving to others you will feel the love you need.

I cannot express enough the personal benefit of being of service to others. But let me put it this way: whether I'm helping an elderly person with their groceries or giving a homeless stranger a smile, doing something for others in need is personally healing. This

"You cannot get through a single day without having an impact on the world around you. What you do makes a difference, and you have to decide what kind of difference you want to make."

—JANE GOODALL

realization came to me one day when I was teaching a Spinning class: I knew that I was a good teacher because, as I looked around the room, I genuinely loved all of my students. I had learned everything about loving from teaching. The love I felt rise up from within me was the love that I was giving. I loved my students for what I could offer them, not for what they were giving to me. It filled me up. It still fills me with emotion to consider this power of service.

The point is: the thing you wish someone would do for you, you can do for another. Of course, you must take care of yourself first. At a certain point during your process—like right now—you must be willing to accept your situation and do everything you can to put the oxygen mask on yourself first, so to speak. You can do this with good self-care habits. (The fact that you're reading this book and have made it to week six indicates that you're on your way.) Then you must be willing to forgo the things you think you want to get, and instead reach out and give to another. That's where the term "let it begin with me" comes into play.

Putting yourself into action toward others will make you happier. Seriously! It's a proven fact: recent studies have shown that people who are of service to others literally raise their own happiness quotient. Trust me, this is great news! It means you don't have to change a thing about your own circumstance, depth of sorrow, or state of mind in order to feel better. To lift your own spirits, you need only reach out to another to lift theirs!

But, like I said, in order to help others you must first fill your own cup with basic self-care. Let's begin with that.

Self-care is not a formula or a checkbox on your to-do list; it represents much more. Self-care is being of service to yourself and recognizing what, exactly, you require. It may take some time to pinpoint the things that serve you best, but it's well worth the search. Don't worry when you veer off track or miss your cues—life will bring you back to your true north through circumstance. Your heart and the ease you feel with it is your compass.

Each time I go through a great loss, I take some time to recalibrate my mental, physical, and emotional health. I know I have to start with the basics: the way I treat my body. I refocus on all the habits that I know are healthy but that I'd stopped doing because I was too busy running around, taking care of others, working, and socializing. As I discussed in Week 1 of this book, during my most recent romantic heartbreak I thought I was practicing self-care, but I found instead that I got to a place where I was very ill. It's not that these habits were bad in and of themselves, but I was depleting myself with no reserve and no support, so the things that had helped in the past were no longer working for me. My beach walks and writing were stifled and my thinking was foggy. I couldn't seem to find my energy. Then, as I was going down for another sleepless and physically uncomfortable night, I got some unexpected clarity. I could feel that the withholding, neglectful, and angry-mother part of my psyche was not willing to help out—and that another part of me needed to step in and get help. Once I got clear that my old conditioning was not serving me, I understood that getting to know and understand my own body in a new way was vital to my healing. Even though I knew so much about health and wellness, I needed to search for what would work for me today. I set out on a quest for more information and, as I uncovered and discovered, I started to learn even more about myself. Armed with knowledge and understanding, I could redefine the healing habits that are right for me. This is true for you, too. It is very important that you stay present and open-minded. Rely on that. From there, find a routine that grounds you in good habits for the next *three to six months*. Being of service and practicing self-care grounded me in the day-to-day and gave me self-esteem. Then I had more to give. That is when I was able to start writing this book and sharing with you.

MY STORY

When my then-friend and soon-to-be-client Jennifer Aniston was going through her divorce, it was divine timing. It followed a series of devastating losses I had recently experienced. It seemed I was taking another major hit every three months: first it was my own breakup. Later, my work relationships suffered a blow when I was fired by the owner of the studio where I'd been successfully teaching for six years. Then I lost my father to lymphoma. Having just gone through the trenches of my own string of tragic losses, I had discovered my own sense of internal strength and experience, which I chose to draw from rather than leaning on the detached concept I'd had prior to that time. Something in my heart compelled me to help Jennifer.

There is an aspect of yoga called *seva*. *Seva* is service. It's what we give back without wanting anything in return. Most organizations and religions have this system built in to their lexicons. It can be called tithing, or donating. You don't have to be religious, belong to a group, or even call it *seva*, but nothing fills your heart like helping another soul can—especially one that is hurting in a way that you can understand and have experienced.

Yes, Jennifer's breakup was very public, but *everyone* can relate to what it feels like when your community knows you're going through heartache and loss. In my neighborhood everyone knew the story of my heartbreak, even if nobody said anything. It was the elephant in the room. There were the mutual friendships that were lost, the move out of our place together, the division of "belongings." Then there were the ex-boyfriend sightings. I seemed to *only* run into my ex or see his car, or walk into a café to find him sitting with a pretty blond girl (his "real" type, I would mutter to myself), at times when I was a zombie in sweatpants.

Because heartbreak is so intensely personal no matter how public the terrain, it can be difficult to be authentic while out in the world. Being honest and vulnerable is so important, yet in public situations we may not always want to open ourselves up to the scrutiny of others. So keeping the focus on where to direct your broken open heart is key. This is where reaching out from your compassionate heart can be a salve. Even when all else fails, you will feel a lot better if you help someone in need because it helps you get out of your own head and into that connection, which you crave.

This week, after you've put your self-care plan into action, be on the lookout for the people in need around you. The antidote to your pain is your ability to share the strength you have gained from a similar experience. If that opportunity does not present itself, there are places that are waiting for you and need you already: the homeless shelter soup kitchen, the hospital children's ward where infants need to be held, the dogs that need walks at the animal shelter. Even a smile to a stranger or going for a walk with an elderly friend is a way to be of service. I call this selfish service because I am the one that benefits from the giving.

Inevitably, when you put yourself out there and do someone a good turn, you gain self-esteem. There's an immediate payoff. All you need to do is be willing and keep your eyes open and reach out when an opportunity presents itself.

SELF-LOVE CHECKLIST

YOGALOSOPHY FOR INNER STRENGTH program

- ☐ **Sunday:** Be Happy Yoga
- ☐ **Monday:** Back-to-Basics Yoga
- ☐ **Tuesday:** Cardio
- ☐ **Wednesday:** Bounce Back! Yoga
- ☐ **Thursday:** Day Off
- ☐ **Friday:** Let Go Yoga
- ☐ **Saturday:** Get Strong Yogalosophy
- ☐ **Heart-Opening Pose:** Heart-Melting Pose
- ☐ **Love Movement:** Active Yoga Class
- ☐ **Heart-Healing Meditation:** Heart Thumping
- ☐ **Love Notes:** Write a Forgiveness Letter
- ☐ **Ritual:** Cleanse
- ☐ **Strength for the Soul:** Practice Self-Care Through Hygiene

MANTRA

I enjoy being in process. It is effortless to take care of myself and it allows me to joyfully help others.

TRACK OF THE WEEK

"Baba Hanuman" by Krishna Das, or "Chamundayai Kali Ma" by Steve Ross

HEART-OPENING POSE: HEART-MELTING POSE

This is a variation on Child's Pose that's also called Extended Puppy Dog Pose. This posture releases tension you may hold in your upper back and expands the front of your body, including the chest and abdominals.

- Begin in Table Top, with wrists below shoulders and knees below hips. Tuck your toes under. Draw your shoulder blades together and pull them down your spine.

- Walk your palms forward and lower your chest slowly, until it is hovering an inch above the ground.
- Gaze ahead about 6 inches and make active contact with the mat through your palms and tucked toes. Hold for 5 to 8 breaths.
- Walk hands back to Table Top to come out of the pose.

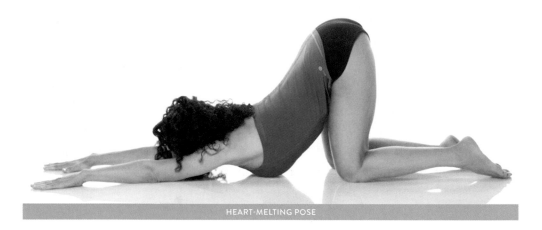

HEART-MELTING POSE

LOVE MOVEMENT: ACTIVE YOGA CLASS

You needn't jump up and down to get your heart rate up. Yoga can be cardiovascular too. Hot yoga will bring the heart rate up because of the high temperature in the room. Vinyasa flow yoga, also called Power Yoga, will get the heart pumping from the continuous flow of movement. Observe how you are feeling physically. While I would love for you to be active, it's essential that you don't deplete yourself—like I did—in your efforts to feel better. Chances are you will be fine to try this for just this one week without any repercussions (remember, my depletion was cumulative and genetic). But note: hot yoga can be deceiving, and the teachers can be rigid at times, so make sure to hydrate before, during, and after class.

Regardless, choose an active yoga class this week. And when you're in the class, imagine that you are serving the other practitioners in the room—by taking supreme care of yourself. This is how we help one another in a group setting.

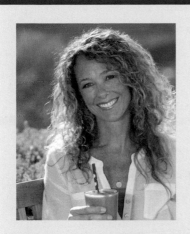

Melissa Costello is the founder of Karma Chow, author of *The Karma Chow Ultimate Cookbook* and *The Clean in 14 Detox*. She also created the "Green" and "Clean" diet options in *Yogalosophy: 28-Days to the Ultimate Mind-Body Makeover* and is a good friend of mine. She provides online cleanses, as well as her guidelines for a physical and emotional cleanse in the Ritual section on pages 247-249. The mind is a reflection of the body, so cleansing the mind of blame and shame are keys to feeling better emotionally and physically. She also offers this week's cleanse-friendly Heart-Healthy Treat on page 253. (For more on her, visit www.KarmaChow.com.)

· · ·

Melissa

Having a broken heart is no fun. Believe me, I've had my share. Sometimes I feel like more than my share, really. There is nothing that can help the pain of a broken heart but time, *and* compassion and kind understanding. In the past, when my heart was broken I reeled in the story of how the other person "did me wrong." I became a victim of my circumstance.

It wasn't until a dear friend gifted me a book, *The Wisdom of a Broken Heart* by Susan Piver, that everything changed. Instead of being a victim and not taking responsibility for myself, I began to practice kind understanding toward myself and my very vulnerable feelings. Instead of hating and blaming the person who broke my heart, I engaged in a daily loving-kindness meditation with him as the focus. I dropped the story and felt the feelings. Boy, was that hard at first, but what I gleaned was that the story I was making up was the most painful part—and not the actual feelings.

Relating to myself with compassion, love, and kindness began the healing process so much more quickly than I had ever experienced in the past. I gave myself permission to feel and not fix. I stopped looking for what was wrong with me and started to take responsibility for how I felt, and what my part had been in the relationship. Making these few small shifts truly set me free, and helped me to keep my heart open instead of shutting down and never wanting to love again.

Look, I know it's never easy to heal from a broken heart, but what you can do is be a whole heck of a lot nicer to yourself as you go through the process, no matter how painful.

HEART-HEALING MEDITATION: HEART THUMPING

Sit and think of someone you really love. Someone who really brings you joy. It can be a child, or someone you care for without needing anything in return. Smile. Make a fist with your hand and pound your chest where your heart is. As you pound your chest say, "Ha ha ha" three times. Do this for three sets of three to activate your heart.

LOVE NOTES: WRITE A FORGIVENESS LETTER

This may be a letter forgiving yourself for what you did not do. It may be a letter forgiving God or the Universal Force for taking away something you love. Or perhaps you may want to write down a list of the things that did not serve you in your broken relationship. This list will serve as a reminder when you have forgotten that feeling in the pit of your stomach. Making a list of what no longer serves you can be a reminder not to move backward. You can reinforce this with some sort of positive affirmation that backs up your releasing the relationship, job, or circumstance.

RITUAL: CLEANSE

Embark on a dietary "cleanse" and notice how your energies are redirected.

ask the expert

CLEANSING AND HOW TO DO IT SIMPLY
BY MELISSA COSTELLO

Cleansing can be scary. When most people hear the word "cleansing" they automatically think starvation and suffering. What I have come to know from my own experience on my lifelong journey with food is that there are ways to cleanse that don't include starvation, drinking a lemon cayenne concoction, or just juicing.

You can cleanse your body by eating food, and a lot of it. Our bodies are incredible and miraculous healing machines that are capable of so much—if we treat them well. I am a huge advocate of food-based cleansing, as detailed in my book *Clean in 14 Detox*. It's all about learning how to eat, and feeling satisfied, which tends to be the opposite of most cleanses.

Our body is the healthiest and works the most optimally when it's in an alkaline state. Our blood must always stay alkaline no matter what, or we would cease to exist. If the body starts to get out of balance and overly acidic—from the ingestion of too much sugar, processed foods, animal products, etc.—the blood has to work really hard to alkalize itself, which means pulling essential nutrients from other areas of the body, such as calcium from the bones. This is usually the start of osteoporosis. So you see, the more alkalizing foods we eat, the more chance we have of our body being a clean, balanced, healthy machine.

You may be wondering where to even start when it comes to food-based cleansing. It can feel overwhelming and confusing. So here are my Top-Five tips on how to gently cleanse your body. This is all about taking baby steps. Try it out for a week and see how you feel. The first few days will be the hardest as your body releases toxins, but you will get over the hump and you will start to feel lighter, brighter, and healthier. Remember, the body will do the work it's meant to when you treat it well. It will function and operate optimally when it receives clean, nutritious food. And if you keep it up, endless possibilities of energy, health, and vitality await you!

MELISSA'S TOP-FIVE CLEANSE TIPS

CUT THE CRAP (SLOW POISON SMACKDOWN):
CRAP a.k.a. Coffee/Caffeine, Refined Sugar, Alcohol, and Processed Foods/Fats. Cutting out these foods/drink for a short period of time will give your body a break and a chance to reset itself. These slow poisons build up in the system and cause inflammation and acid. Remember, we want alkaline! Add plenty of fruits, veggies, nuts, seeds, whole grains, beans, and lean proteins to your diet. During this time be sure to eat only whole foods—nothing that comes in a bag, box, or can. Check out the recipe on page 253 for detox deliciousness. You won't even believe it's cleanse-friendly.

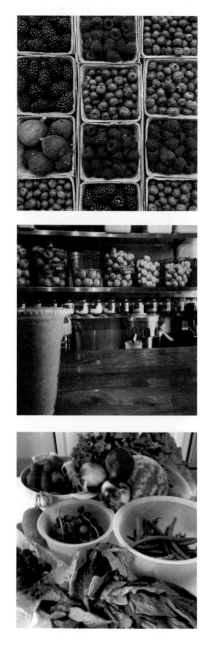

DRINK PLENTY OF WATER: Water is extremely essential for the body and helps flush toxins out of the system. You want to drink at least half an ounce of water for every pound of your body weight. You can drink more if you so desire, as it will help you in flushing out your internal organs and keeping your digestive system working optimally.

SLEEP AND REST: I am always blown away when my clients tell me they get only five or six hours of sleep per night. Sleep is essential to our health and well-being. Our body detoxes and repairs at night when we are in a deep sleep state. It's important to build a ritual around sleep and do your best to go to bed at the same time every night—and unplug from all electronics at least an hour, if not more, before going to bed. This will ensure a deeper, more restful sleep.

MOVE YOUR BODY: Exercise is important when you're detoxing. It's best to engage in gentle movement such as yoga, cycling, dance, walking, swimming, etc., for a minimum of 20 to 30 minutes per day. This will assist your body in flushing toxins and keeping your metabolism firing for maximum results.

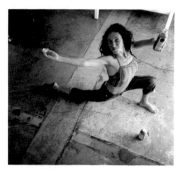

EAT WITH AWARENESS: You are busy, I get that, but it's almost impossible to have a healthy body if you are constantly eating on the go. It wreaks havoc on the digestive system. When you eat a meal, sit down, chew your food, enjoy the flavors, put your fork down in between bites, and practice gratitude for the food and nutrition that is on your plate.

• • •

A shift in diet may not be what works best for you. There are other ways to restrict habitual behaviors in favor of new, healthier ways of being. You could try a media detox: eliminate TV, computer, the Internet (no email, no Facebook!), and radio —take a week to allow your mind to get clear, with no input from the outside. If you feel you can't media detox because of work or obligations, limit yourself to no Internet or television after 6:00 PM. Observe what other activities arise from this restriction.

Decide what you are willing to let go of for a week. I even selected one musical album ("PRANA," by Shaman's Dream) that felt neutral to me, and I would listen to it over and over again just to be soothed. (My next-door neighbor may have gone crazy!) Because I played it incessantly, each time I revisit the album I become increasingly relaxed and at ease. Find what works for you.

STRENGTH FOR THE SOUL: PRACTICE SELF-CARE THROUGH HYGIENE

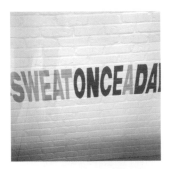

MOUTH: flossing, dental exam (teeth cleaning), tongue scraping, coconut oil pulling (swish 1–2 teaspoons of coconut oil in your mouth for 20 minutes. Spit out— *do not swallow*—as it has pulled toxins from your body. Rinse well with warm water and brush your teeth and tongue.)

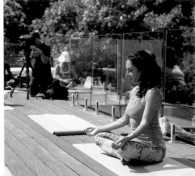

HAIR: haircut, deep conditioning

FACE: mask, revamping cleansing regime

BODY: dry brush massage, self-massage, professional massage, infrared sauna, Epsom salt bath

DIET/DIGESTION: shifting your diet, elimination diet, fasting, liver flush, colonic, coffee enema

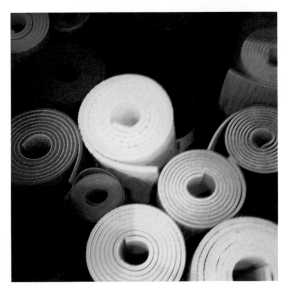

MEDICAL: checkup, OB/GYN, mammogram, blood work

HANDS-ON HEALING: acupuncture, chiropractic, cranial/sacral, body work, reiki

SUPPLEMENTS: aloe juice, Cal-Mag powder, herbs, probiotics, apple cider vinegar drink (32 ounces water, 4 tablespoons Bragg's Apple Cider Vinegar, 4 tablespoons lemon juice, 1 teaspoon ground cinnamon, 4 tablespoons raw honey: Dissolve cinnamon, lemon, and honey in hot water, stir well. Add Apple Cider Vinegar. Enjoy hot or cold.)

GENERAL SOOTHERS: walking, castor oil packs, hot water bottle, lemon in warm water

 The human heart is the size of a large fist, weighs between 10 and 12 ounces, and beats 100,000 times per day.

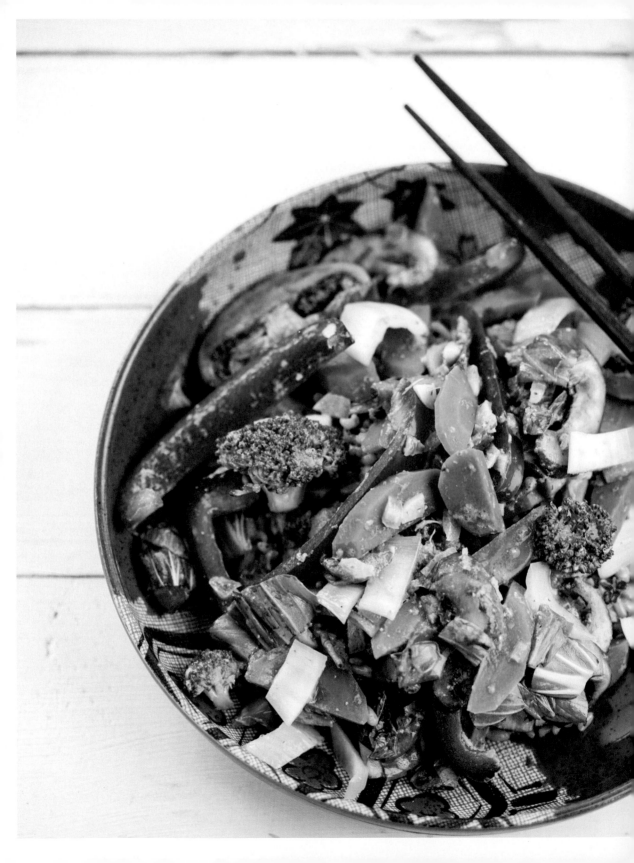

COCONUT BASIL STIR FRY

Serves 4

This hearty dish is completely vegan and will satisfy your taste buds and your tummy without the heaviness. A wonderful meal if you want to try for a Meatless Monday. This is not your typical stir-fry—the flavors from the basil and the coconut milk seem to elevate it to a whole new level of deliciousness!

SAUCE INGREDIENTS

1 CUP FRESH BASIL LEAVES

1 CUP REGULAR FULL-FAT COCONUT MILK

2 TABLESPOONS BRAGG'S LIQUID AMINOS

1 TABLESPOON FRESH LEMON JUICE

2 TEASPOONS RICE VINEGAR

1 TEASPOON ARROWROOT POWDER (THICKENER)

1 TABLESPOON GRADE B MAPLE SYRUP OR COCONUT SUGAR

STIR FRY INGREDIENTS

1 TABLESPOON COCONUT OIL

2 CLOVES GARLIC, MINCED

1/4 CUP DICED RED ONION

1 TEASPOON GRATED FRESH GINGER

4 MEDIUM CARROTS, HALVED AND CUT INTO 1/4-INCH DIAGONAL SLICES

1 RED BELL PEPPER, DESEEDED AND CUT INTO STRIPS

1 CUP THINLY SLICED MUSHROOMS

1 CUP BROCCOLI FLORETS

1 CUP THINLY SLICED BOK CHOY OR CABBAGE

3 CARROTS, HALVED AND DICED

1 CUP COOKED QUINOA OR BROWN RICE

Put the coconut sauce ingredients in a blender and blend to combine. Set aside.

To prepare the stir-fry, heat the oil in a large wok or sauté pan over medium-high heat. Sauté the garlic, onion, and ginger until soft. Add the carrots, bell pepper, and mushrooms. Cook for another 3 minutes. Add the broccoli and bok choy. Stir to combine.

Pour the coconut sauce over the veggies and cover the pan with a lid. Decrease heat to medium. Stirring occasionally, let the veggies steam in the sauce for a few minutes until the sauce begins to thicken. Do not overcook the veggies or let them get soggy. Serve over quinoa or brown rice.

Recipe by Melissa Costello

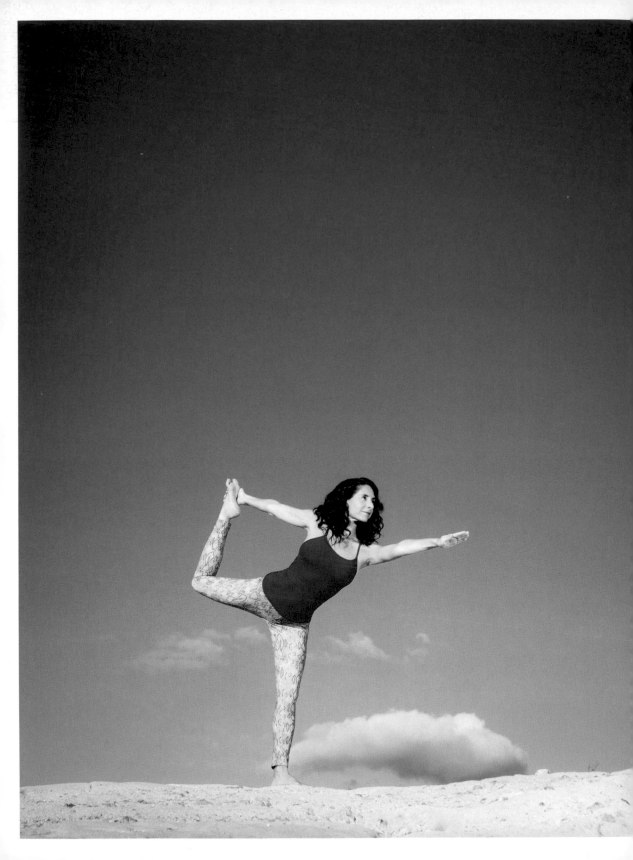

WEEK 7

Bounce Back to Balance and Beauty

You have no control over what other people do, feel, or say. You can't make someone love you when they don't, will a sick or dying loved one back to vitality, or change the painful or unkind behavior of others. The only hope you have of making a major change in your life is to take the focus off others and put it back on *you*. That's why this week we're going to put down the magnifying glass and pick up the mirror.

Let me explain. In any story or situation that involves someone else, you have control over only your half of it. You cannot stand in, direct, or change the course of another person's journey. But most of us can't help but try, especially when we desperately want something. So, often our half of the story is spent giving the other person the power—by wishing *they* were different, or wanting or trying to control the outcome of life's twists and turns rather than focusing on creating a better life for ourselves. But here's the thing: when you look to another to provide what you can actually give to yourself, you can become dependent and out of practice to the point that you forget your power—not to mention that you can become the passenger rather than the driver in your own life. You cannot do anything to change the course of your story unless you *see* it differently. But if you shift yourself and focus on your 50 percent, the world will magically fall into place around you and your life will get 100 percent better!

> "As human beings, our greatness lies not so much in being able to remake the world . . . [but] in being able to remake ourselves."
>
> —MAHATMA GANDHI

When you recognize that you don't have to "have it all together," and that the universe is a big place, with room for all sorts of possibilities, you broaden your world. And that is just as well, because when you take a look at yourself and what you *do* have control over—your behaviors, your mind, the actions you take—all possibilities open up.

Let's take as an example the case of being fired. We all know that there's no use in working for someone who doesn't feel you're beneficial to them. Yet, the pain of rejection, fear of the unknown, and loss of security can feel overwhelming, and your 50 percent can easily be spent immersed in self-pity—as well as in behavior that keeps you there. However, while you may not be able to call the shots, you do have choices. Specifically, you can choose to embrace the lessons learned through your experience and give yourself a mental makeover.

Easier said than done, right? Maybe not. The first thing you need to do is reframe your loss as beneficial to you. Rather than focusing on how painful the situation is or how disappointing someone has been, you can *choose* to feel grateful and blessed by the situation because it is bringing you to a new level of strength and self-awareness. Once you've done that, you can redirect the energy you may have been spending trying to get something from another to instead focus squarely on what you can give to yourself.

You may be saying: "My situation is different. My pain is greater than this. My circumstance cannot be fixed. Life will never be the same again." Let me tell you, I completely understand. After my father's early death at age sixty, I felt sad that things would never be the same. I am the eldest of his four children and was able to resolve my issues with him prior to his passing—but that was not the case for his other children, particularly his younger set. My half-siblings, at age twelve and ten, were too young to process the loss. In my experience, death causes different reactions to the ones left behind. Someone once told me that people die as they have lived, and my father was quite complicated. Although he was surrounded by love, he left a lot of turmoil behind in his wake.

After having lost touch with my youngest brother, I found out several years later that he'd had a psychotic break and was diagnosed with schizophrenia. When I first found out I was devastated beyond compare, and wracked with guilt that I had not been there for him enough to help support him. My heart was remorseful and I felt ashamed. I did not know what to do.

When I shared with a trusted friend how I was feeling, she suggested that I simply reach out to him and let him know I was thinking of him. I mustered the courage to send him a birthday gift through my half-sister, Megan, with whom I'd maintained a connection. After she gave the gift to him, she said he mentioned he would like to be in touch. I gave him a call, and to my surprise, the tiny action of my reaching out was enough for him. When I told him I was sorry I had not been in touch, he immediately let me know it was okay. His generosity and politeness humbled me to tears.

Since that day we've remained in contact, and he now has a strong support group. I trust that he is being taken care of by a guiding force, as well as by a host of helpers who are giving him what he needs. I am especially moved by the male authority figures that are helping to guide him daily, for he lacked that cornerstone in his youth. I try to remember that I am here for him when he needs me, and that I am not in charge of his life. Everything worked out.

To get in the right mind-set for detaching, I recommend drawing an imaginary circle around your body and reminding yourself that everything within the circle is all that you are really in charge of—and that it's plenty. Everything you need to find the beauty and balance in your life is contained within that circle, and you have complete control over it. You can and will bounce back to your own circle and your own, now greater, sense of personal power.

MY STORY

When I woke up this morning to write, I felt I'd been in a two-day fog. I'd been wishing and fantasizing and even obsessing on a work project that I really wanted to happen, but that didn't work out. I went down the rabbit hole of thought, and gracefully came out the other side today. I can feel a change in my thinking. There is an antidote I like that applies: in Chinese medicine or in Ayurvedic health systems, the elements are considered part of health imbalances. For instance, the mind is connected to the air element. When the air element is imbalanced, one thinks too much and talks too much. Air needs fire, which is activated and directed by creativity. So I can take the direct "fire" action of writing a chapter of this book. As I write, the Shaman's Dream album "PRANA" is playing (the one I shared about in the last chapter). There are no lyrics, just music. I am sipping warm water with lemon to help my digestion, as I know I want to soothe and gently cleanse myself. It's 7:30 AM. I skipped morning meditation, as felt I wanted to jump right in with you as a part of my meditation. I have rebounded from the constraints of "what I want" into the humility of "I want what the universe wants for me." I accept what is, and I can do something productive with it. Of course it would be nice if another person came into the picture and told me that I had the deal I was looking for and gave me a big fat contract to sign—but I have what I need in this moment. And anyway, if that did occur I would not be strengthening my experience of faith as I am now.

Then there are things you *can* do. There are ways to work around this. How many times have you sat waiting for that raise, for that love note, for the other person to help with the dishes or the grocery bill . . . or to give you a gift? But what if you didn't "wait"? What if you did for yourself what you are waiting for others to do for you? It's good to practice giving to the self. Many of us have been raised to downplay our own needs or think it's selfish to give to ourselves. My mother never bought herself anything new, and that influenced me a lot, in the reverse-psychology way. I always wondered why she put herself last. I did not view this as an amazing sacrifice she was making for me, especially since every once in a while she would explode with rage and list out all the things she'd done for me. Resentfully making a list of your sacrifices will not serve anybody, especially yourself. It's time to put down that list, and make a new one: the list of what you can give to yourself! Remind yourself with little gestures that you deserve to have beauty and you, in fact, are the love of your life!

This week, take extra time to love what you see in the mirror. Each situation and human is a direct reflection of something within yourself. So, loving it all is a key to loving yourself. I remember a couple I knew who said that "nothing was sacred" and that was how they kept their relationship honest. At first, I did not comprehend what that meant. When I thought about it later, I realized that this meant they had no secrets. They accepted everything and turned over every stone to find the beauty in all of it. When you look in the mirror, see all of your beauty. When you see the world, see yourself.

Do a full 30 minutes of cardio on your rebounder to reinforce that mentality of bouncing back to your natural state of health and beauty.

PERSEPHENIE'S STORY

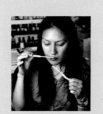

My longtime friend Persephenie Lea is a Los Angeles–based artist, certified aromatherapist, and perfumer specializing in natural botanical perfumery. Persephenie formulates and produces her line of body and face care, perfumes, incenses, and aromatic candies. She prides herself in using carefully selected materials and not using heavy preservatives. She thinks of her studio as an Old World aromatic apothecary, or a place to satiate olfactory wanderlust where sundries and therapeutics are meticulously crafted. Find her Heart Beauty Treatments in the Heart Connection section on page 264.

• • •

Persephenie

When I met Solomon, he was wearing diapers and sitting on the counter of my father's store. He was tiny, barely two, and full of life. Solomon's mom worked for my father, and over the next few years Solomon and his mom integrated into our family. My parents thought of Solomon and his mom as their own. His mom became my sister, and Solomon their grandson. Significant milestones for Solomon were important: birthdays, shows, Halloween costumes, family celebrations, and shared holidays.

Shortly after my son's third birthday, Solomon was killed. He was a healthy nine-year-old boy, maturing, funny, smart, on the edge of embracing a double-digit number, and the possibilities were wide open for him. It felt unfair. His death was unfathomable and unacceptable. The weight and pain on my heart was overwhelming, and the people I loved suffered with me. I had felt heartache from loss before, but the finality and circumstances of his death, coupled with his age and with being a new mom myself—well, the term "heartbreak" feels like an understatement.

It took time and a lot of work to let go. I can give credit to grief and the need to heal for sparking my interest in essential oils as a tool for handling sadness. To smell, to breathe in life again, to get out of my head, and to be in the present through scent was incredibly healing.

HEART-HEALING MEDITATION: SELF-GAZING

Sit in front of a mirror and gaze into your own eyes. Breathe and connect with your heart. Do not lose eye contact with yourself. Say, "I love you." Repeat over and over again for 5 minutes. This is a lot more challenging than it sounds. It is also way more effective than you realize. Try it and see what you find.

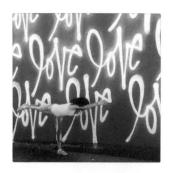

LOVE NOTES:
WHAT DO YOU WANT IN ANOTHER?

Make a list of the qualities you would want in a partner. How many of these qualities do you embody yourself? Can you become those qualities? If you became more of this for yourself and others, would you even require this from your partner at all? One of the primary needs that I recognized in this most recent breakup period is that I want someone who has time for me. I soon recognized that I make very little time for myself. Or, at least I need a lot more time, and for someone—me!—to take a real interest. I followed suit, cleared my decks, and have made more space for myself. It works. All sorts of new desires and creations are bubbling up and I feel loved.

RITUAL: CREATE A VISION BOARD
OF WHAT YOU LOVE

Even after my ex and I had broken up, I saved my "love and marriage" vision board for a while, thinking that this breakup may have been part of the journey to my receiving all of these visions for myself. After a short time, I knew I had to revisit this board. Did it

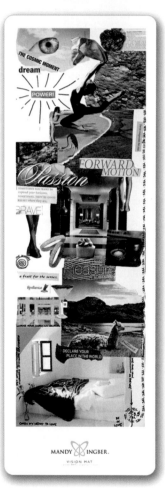

THIS PHOTO AND OPPOSITE © JENNIFER CAWLEY

really represent me? Or was this an attempt to save the relationship and keep it intact? As I viewed it with soft focus, it just felt so busy. It seemed confusing and did not have the clarity, focus, and simplicity that I crave in my heart.

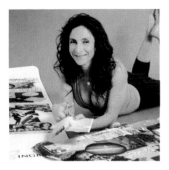

I had seen a few images in the past that looked like what I really wanted in a relationship. I pulled these three images from the Internet. I printed them and placed them on my poster board: the simplicity of Alex Grey's *lovers' electricity*, representing connectedness and passion; the friendship, romance, and togetherness of the silhouetted hand-holding of a couple at sunset; and the spiritual, conscious, universal love of the drawing of a couple connected at the crown and mind, which includes a quote from Ram Dass: "Real love is the One celebrating itself as the Two." After I glued these images, whose clarity evoke a deep feeling in me, I also arranged qualities or words around them. I claim the love that I am gravitating toward with this visual, emotion-evoking love-vision board.

So, this week, create a vision board of what you love, or what makes your heart sing.

STRENGTH FOR THE SOUL: WAYS TO PAMPER YOURSELF

Waxing	Facial	Natural products facial mask
Electrolysis	Manicure	Flower essence remedy
Day spa	Pedicure	Blow dry bar
Luxury vacation	Body scrub	Mud baths
Retreat	Eyebrow tweeze	V-steam
Visit a perfumery	Hot oil treatment	Korean spa
Find a new scent	Salve from coconut oil	

ask the expert

HEART BEAUTY TREATMENTS: ESSENTIAL OILS AND HEART MASKS BY PERSEPHENIE LEA

1. DIRECT INHALATION

In a meditative position, place one drop of essential oil in the palm of your hands and inhale. Feel the oil work through your lungs and throughout your body. Relax, breathe deeply, and inhale again as needed. For invigoration, use basil or peppermint. For a calm uplift, try bergamot or Melissa oil. For a meditative state, use frankincense.

2. MASSAGE HEART OIL

Flower oils are known to open the heart and clear stagnation. Add 15 drops of a flower essential oil into a half of an ounce of a carrier oil and rub on your heart whenever needed. Try a botanical neroli, rose, or jasmine as your flower oil, and almond or apricot as your carrier oil.

3. HEART-CLEANSING MASK

For the weight of heartache, a series of heart cleanses feels soothing. Using a simple clay like bentonite or French green clay, add water to make a paste. Spread a thin layer of paste on your chest, heart, and breasts. Be in a comfortable temperature where you can be topless as you let the paste dry for 10 to 15 minutes. Open the chest and try direct inhalation with an essential oil. To rinse off you can shower or bathe, or remove with a warm, wet washcloth. Afterward, massage your heart with your Massage Heart Oil.

HEART FACT — In a 2005 study of the brain and heartbreak, subjects who were hooked up to an MRI scanner showed that the part of the brain that is activated from a broken heart is the same part of the brain that registers physical pain. This is part of why heartbreak hurts so much.

RADIANT SWEET POTATO AND BUTTERNUT SQUASH SOUP

Serves 4—6

This thick and creamy soup is dairy-free and filled with flavor. It is chock-full of potassium and fiber and is low calorie (only 82 calories per cup!). Potassium is known for preventing high blood pressure, so this filling dish will go a long way to slow you down. Vitamin A is key to great skin as it will keep you moisturized. Fiber will keep it all moving. A comfort food to enjoy, guilt free!

SPICE PASTE

2 TABLESPOONS CORIANDER

2 TABLESPOONS FENNEL SEEDS

4 TEASPOONS OREGANO

1 TEASPOON CHILI FLAKES

1 TEASPOON HIMALAYAN
    PINK SALT

1 TEASPOON PEPPER

4 TABLESPOONS OLIVE OIL

SOUP FIXINS

3 LARGE SWEET POTATOES, PEELED AND CUT INTO
    WEDGES

1½ BUTTERNUT SQUASH, CUT IN 3-INCH-THICK
    WEDGES

2 TABLESPOONS COCONUT OIL

2 ONIONS, CHOPPED

1 INCH GINGER, GRATED

4 CUPS VEGETABLE STOCK

1 CAN COCONUT MILK

2 TABLESPOONS MAPLE SYRUP

Preheat oven to 200°F. Combine all the spice paste ingredients in a small bowl and set aside.

Line two baking trays with parchment paper.

Rub the sweet potatoes and squash with the spice paste. Place them on the baking trays and bake for 40 minutes.

Put the coconut oil and onions in a large pot over medium heat and stir them together. When the onions become translucent, add the ginger. After taking the sweet potatoes and squash out of the oven, add the sweet potato to the pot and stir. (Set aside the squash to cool a bit.) Add the vegetable stock and stir. Once the squash is cool enough to touch, peel away the skin and chop the flesh, adding to the pot as you go.

Blend the soup (with an immersion blender or high-powered heat-safe blender) until smooth. Add the coconut milk, maple syrup, and salt and pepper to taste.

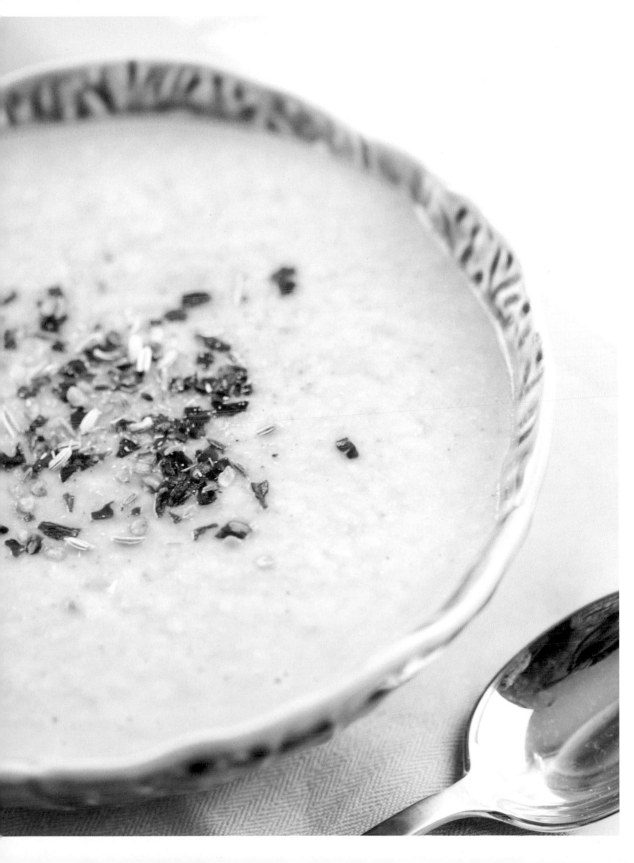

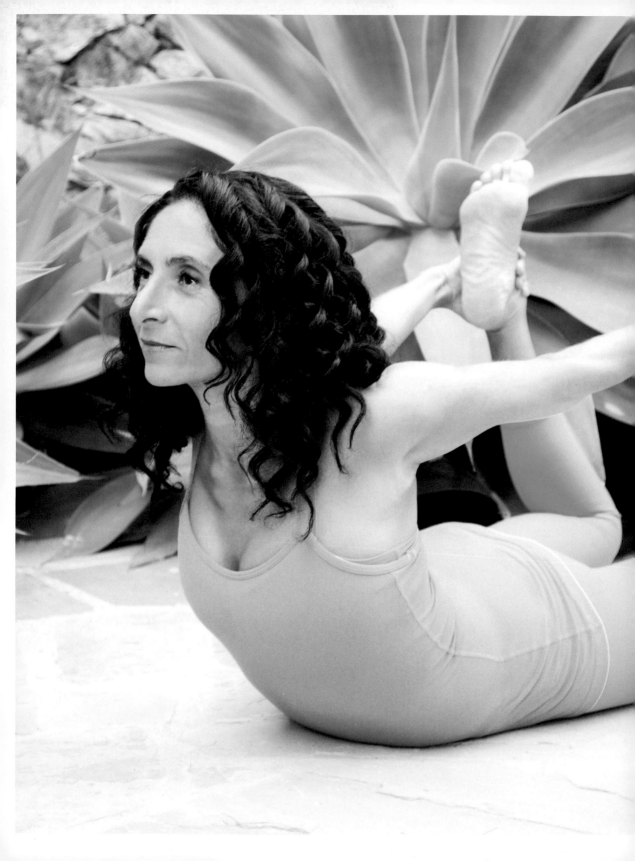

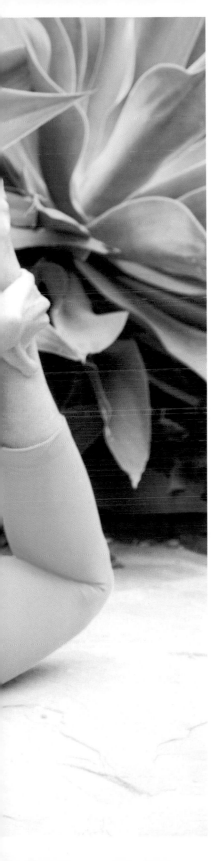

WEEK 8

Flirt with Life

This week we're going to explore intimacy. I don't mean your relationship with another. I'm talking about intimacy with yourself: getting to know and embrace the things about you that you hide or deny because they may not seem as appealing to you as some of your other attributes. And getting up close and personal with your sexuality and sensual side. There are good reasons to get excited about this exploration. You'll find that in getting to  know your shadow side, you'll not only feel more self-confident, you'll also discover that what you set aside, denied, or hid from sight is actually what is truly special and most lovably human about you.

True intimacy with yourself and with others comes from going deeper to experience the world's impact on you—what inspires, injures, or incenses you—and also taking in *your* effect on your world, and sharing that honestly. It's a special state when you're beyond the illusion of the duality of good and evil, of right and wrong, and instead are dancing with life itself in its myriad of colors, its depth, and its heights.

Taking the time to uncover, decode, and explore your depth is not always celebrated in our fast-paced culture. Discovering the shadow can be unpopular because most people like to present themselves as a perfect package, as "looking good," and intimacy is really messy. It's also the most exquisite aspect of life, which allows you to be seen for all of who you are, including the light, ethereal, subtle part of your human self as well as your inadequacies, caverns of pain, and the traumas that tinge your ability to openly receive from others and the world around you. Our most intimate aspects are those that usually hide in the shadow. But when revealed, they're healed simply by their exposure; standing as your authentic self, you will find that the truth does indeed set you free.

Intimacy is what I crave the most and resist the hardest. I forget my true core, and my slower, deeper rhythm, and mask it with my persona. In examining this pattern, I ward an intimacy with the self. This requires nothing of the folks nething I am able to explore alone. The same is true for you. acy as something that only exists between two people. But you your own right. Now is the time to get to know yourself in a nd yes, that includes sexuality. st losses when we lose romantic love is the intimacy that comes as with all else, you can be self-reliant in this way, too. There are s, and even ruts that we adopt when we are in an intimate physi- a lover. It's in this physical realm that we create bonding, and our sexual space can become a world of its own that's almost like a magical ritual. When you've lost that connection or bond, it's time to return to yourself and create your own pleasurable, magical space.

There's not one right way to do that. The question is: what works for you? Often we play into only certain aspects of sexuality, sometimes out of inhibition, laziness, or being shy with our partner. This is a time to open up again and explore your sexuality.

Just begin by becoming more truthful, sensual, and opening up to the feeling of sexuality as you walk through the world will activate this exploration. It could be a way that you dress, a person you flirt with (or noticing someone is flirting with you), or even just a curiosity you entertain. It could be allowing someone to see something about you that you think is best kept under wraps. Pay attention to the things that excite you in this present moment. No need to do anything about it; in fact, let it come to you.

❀ MY STORY

Attraction is like a magnet. You don't need to conquer anything. Just allow the play of the exchange between you and your surroundings to affect you, and notice your effect. It's okay to get curious about your own sexuality. Sexuality can heal more than just a breakup; it is the rawness of your grief that can open you up to being truly seen. I remember one period when I opened myself up to being more flirtatious. I was twenty-seven, and still an actress. I had shot a pilot, a prototype for a television show. Pilots either get picked up and made into a series, or not. This was a "not," but one thing I did pick up on was an attraction to one of my costars. Let's call him Kenny, since his name was Kenny. By the time we were shooting the show a week had passed, which had provided enough time in one another's presence for me to develop a healthy crush. He, being the flirt that he was, seemed to have a crush on another girl as well. At first I was disappointed when I walked into the rehearsal on set to see this cute redhead sitting right next to my crush. I hesitated, but then I let my flirty self take over. If I felt excluded, why didn't I just go sit next to him on the other side? So I did. Later that night, I was sitting alone backstage and meditating prior to filming. (Note to the yogis and yoginis: meditation doesn't belong to just you! It is not uncommon for actors to incorporate meditation prior to a performance to reduce anxiety and get relaxed, centered, and open.) Something caused me to open my eyes, and there was Kenny. Surprised to see me, he almost left. Then I said, "I willed you here." (This is my subtle version of flirting.) Anyway, it worked . . . if you call a three-month fling, wherein he started seeing one of my friends at the tail end of our relationship, something that worked. Sigh. Yes, flirting with life can be fun if you keep the focus on yourself. After that chapter, I flung myself into a new career as a Spinning instructor, and the next guy I met was "the one" . . . for a while.

Here's how I started finding the confidence to flirt, and here's a suggestion for you: imagine seeing yourself across a crowded room, and begin a flirtation that grows deeper as you learn more about you. Access the dark and the light, the ways you are strong and the ways you are devastated. Explore and examine who you are in every respect. Grief and a broken heart is really an opening for accessing this depth. This is where all the juicy stuff lives. Don't be afraid to feel around in the dark. In my public classes, I find that when awareness about shame is raised, seen, and named—and even laughed about—a lightness opens up in the room. The very naming and witnessing is the healing power itself. I also talked about sex in my class, which didn't hurt either.

This week, love your darkness and your shadow side! Yoga honors the dark and the light. We all have stuff. We have things we feel are shameful or imagine that only we feel. The obsessions, the jealousy, and the despairing broken heart are a part of who you are. There is even a power and a magic at the center of these depths. Underneath the surface, something is hidden that calls to you. Shine a light on it with the truth and watch what transforms.

SELF-LOVE CHECKLIST
YOGALOSOPHY FOR INNER STRENGTH program
- ☐ **Sunday:** Be Happy Yoga
- ☐ **Monday:** Back-to-Basics Yoga
- ☐ **Tuesday:** Cardio
- ☐ **Wednesday:** Bounce Back! Yoga
- ☐ **Thursday:** Day Off
- ☐ **Friday:** Let Go Yoga
- ☐ **Saturday:** Get Strong Yogalosophy
- ☐ **Heart-Opening Pose:** Bow
- ☐ **Love Movement:** Weight Training
- ☐ **Heart-Healing Meditation:** Goddess Durga Meditation
- ☐ **Love Notes:** Write Your Feminine Power Fantasy
- ☐ **Ritual:** Create an Altar to the Mystery
- ☐ **Strength for the Soul:** Sensual Pleasures

MANTRA

I am transforming into the person that is the highest vibration of myself. I am a sexual, intimate, vibrant being.

TRACK OF THE WEEK

Sexy song: "Erotic City" by Prince. Ultimate longing song: "Moonlight Mile" by The Rolling Stones. All-time favorite revenge song: "Your Time Is Gonna Come" by Led Zeppelin. (Other notable tracks: "The Weight" by The Band, or "Eye of the Tiger" by Survivor.)

HEART-OPENING POSE: BOW

- Begin on your belly with your forehead resting on the mat, your arms down by your sides. Take 3 long, deep breaths.

- Resting your chin on the floor, bend your knees and bring your heels toward your butt. Reach back and grip the tops of your feet or ankles (with your hands on the outsides, not insides, of your feet).

- Gaze straight ahead. Take a deep breath in. On the exhale, lift your shoulders, legs, and torso off the floor.

- Draw your shoulder blades down your back and breathe.

- After 3 to 5 deep breaths, slowly lower your body back to the floor and rest your head to one side. Repeat 3 times.

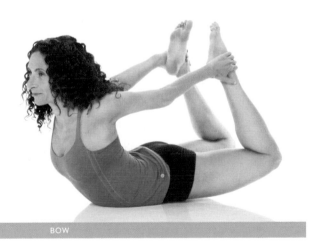

BOW

LOVE MOVEMENT: WEIGHT TRAINING

Lift your heart, strengthen your bones, and build your intimacy with the self by working past your edge. Weight training is another option for making your heart healthy. It strengthens blood vessels and makes your heart strong. Other benefits include regulating blood pressure and cholesterol. The routine needs to be of adequate intensity, so if you have a trainer or go to a gym,

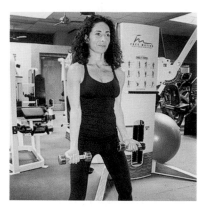

get there this week, or seek out a weight training group class. Yes, you may need to go the extra mile to find it, but that's exactly what this week is all about. While you're at it . . . wear something that makes you feel sexy—and work it!

LAURA'S STORY

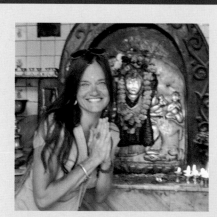

I have asked my dear friend Laura Amazzone, priestess, intuitive, and author of *Goddess Durga and Sacred Female Power*, to share a healing meditation to aid with loss that cannot be repaired. The meditation can be found on pages 276 and 277. Here she shares a story of losing her spiritual home that is both universal and personal.

• • •

Laura

I had never grieved a physical place before, but when a 7.8 earthquake struck Nepal on April 25, 2015, I felt as if my heart and soul were as crushed as the destruction I was witnessing in my beloved spiritual home. In the days that followed, the magnitude of the devastation became more and more shocking and apparent. Entire villages were wiped out, over eight thousand people lost their lives, and thousands of others were left injured, orphaned, and homeless. The weight of the suffering has been unbearable.

The earthquake also destroyed much of the rich cultural and spiritual architectural heritage to which I have devoted my life and work for the past two decades.

One of the things I love most about Nepal is paying homage to and meditating at these sacred sites that devotees, pilgrims, and seekers like myself had visited on a daily basis over millennia. Suddenly, in an instant so much of what I loved, not only people I knew, but also the temples and shrines I had visited countless times, were 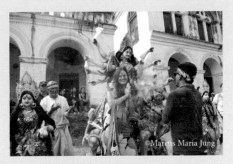 gone. These were sacred places where I had whispered some of my most intimate concerns, fears, hopes, and desires to the goddesses housed there. For days I cried at the thought that I would never again see them or so many other places I loved.

Being in California and so far away from Nepal, I felt helpless and overwhelmed by grief. For the first week after the earthquake I could hardly leave my bed. In my sadness, all I could do was pray and turn to the Goddess Durga, a goddess who had first been introduced to me in Nepal, and who I had been taught to call on in times of great heartbreak and loss. Meditating on and chanting to Durga has helped me to move through this challenging time and the heartbreak I am experiencing. While the Nepal I knew and loved will never be the same, when I focus on Durga, I know that the refuge I found in Nepal can always be found in my heart.

ask the expert

HEART-HEALING MEDITATION:
GODDESS DURGA MEDITATION
BY LAURA AMAZZONE

Durga is a South Asian goddess who helps us transform and release difficult emotions like grief and sadness. She is a goddess of strength and courage who for thousands of years has been known to remove fear, sorrow, and difficulty. One of the meanings of her name is "fortress." This "fortress" refers to the spiritual, emotional, and mental protection She offers to our hearts and minds. Durga is sometimes described as the "eye of the storm." She is that place of calm in the center of chaos. When we invoke Her energies through meditation, visualization, and chanting, we can take refuge in the calmness She offers—even in the midst of the unruly emotions an experience like devastation can bring.

We can call on Durga to teach us about the invincibility of our hearts and to help us find a sense of balance and peace within. When we tune into Her divine essence, Durga reminds us of our strength and gently helps us find the courage to consciously approach and release our fears and sorrows. Durga will always lead us back to the sanctuary of our hearts and remind us that, no matter how difficult our situation may be, there is always much wisdom and insight to be gained from our experience. She teaches us to allow our anguish to become an opportunity to be more compassionate and loving toward our self.

MEDITATION ON DURGA

Sit comfortably and close your eyes. Take a few deep breaths and tune into your body and heart. Bring your focus to the base of your spine and imagine a trunk of a tree with great roots extending down from the base of your body and connecting into the Earth. Feel any sadness, pain, heaviness, or tension releasing down the grounding cord and returning to the Earth. Allow yourself to let go and use your breath to help you find your center. Slowly bring your awareness to your third eye, which is located in the space between the eyebrows. Notice any energy there as you bring your awareness to it. If you feel any discomfort, see that energy releasing down your grounding cord. When you are ready, and with your eyes still closed, shift your focus to about a foot out in front of you and imagine a screen appearing there. On that screen is the Goddess Durga seated astride Her tiger, wearing red and gold, adorned with jewels and flowers and smiling. She appears calm and composed and Her countenance exudes the compassion She feels for all Her children. She appears to alleviate our suffering. In Her eighteen arms and hands She holds various tools and weapons, including a sword to sever toxic attachments, a bell for clarity, a bow and arrow for focus, a spear for penetrating insight, and a shield for protection.

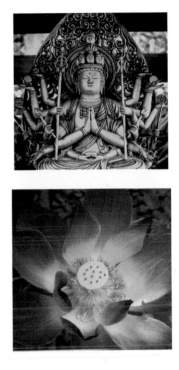

Continue to witness the Goddess Durga before you and allow Her love and compassion to stream from Her heart to yours. As you keep the vision, slowly begin to chant Durga's mantra: "*Aum Dhum* (pronounced "doom") *Durgayay Namaha.*" The vibrations created by this mantra help dispel fear, grief, pain, and difficulty. They bring balance and equilibrium to the mind and heart. Chant as long as you feel comfortable.

When you complete the mantra, continue to visualize Durga before you and offer Her your fears and sadness. Share the prayers of your heart with Her. After a few minutes you may want to ask Her to offer you a tool to help you in your grieving process. What do you need to help you come back to your center and feel at peace? Reflect on what She offers and how you feel about it. How can you apply this tool in your own life? If the answer does not come immediately, you may become more aware of its meaning in the coming days. Look for synchronicities! Ask Her if there is anything else you need to know and see what arises. Maybe you hear a faint or loud voice inside, or perhaps She offers you something else. Trust what your intuition receives. Feel the compassion and love of Durga in your heart, and express your gratitude and anything else you wish to share. When this exchange feels complete, take a deep breath and watch Her image before you dissolving as you breathe Her into your heart. Keep your awareness on your heart center for a few breaths, knowing this is a safe, healing, and calm refuge to which you can always return.

LOVE NOTES: WRITE YOUR
FEMININE POWER FANTASY

Write out a fantasy of your female power or your own version of erotica. Anything goes. Make it really steamy and detailed and handwrite this in your journal or create a myth wherein you inhabit the goddess. This is for you alone, so no holds barred. Many of us ignore this powerful aspect of ourselves, giving no special attention to this pleasure center that is vital to our health, well-being, and happiness. Sexuality is at the root of feminine power—after all, we can create entire villages of people with this energy! Take the time this week to indulge in your sexuality. Turn yourself on!

RITUAL:
CREATE AN ALTAR TO THE MYSTERY

Create an altar to the mystery, the deep side of yourself. It should or can include the destructive aspect of yourself, your sexuality, your anger, the part of you that gives up, the imposter. It should include the depth of your spirit, a primal part of yourself, and the aspect of you that survives and rises to the top no matter what. The parts of you that you don't act out or that you don't share with others. In the Hindu tradition, there are many faces of god/goddess, and they all get to come to the altar to be honored. Just as Laura spoke of the goddess Durga, there are many symbols of her, like the goddess Kali who destroys in order to re-create. It never escapes me that I need to have a dancing Shiva on my altar. The lord Shiva is part of a triad: Brahma (the creator), Vishnu (the preserver), and Shiva—the force of destruction or, rather, rebirth. Restructuring and creating anew from

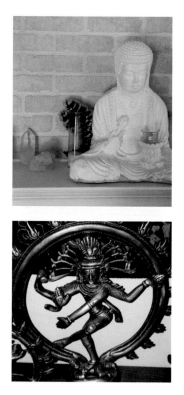

what once was. This is a perfect symbol for me, since often when I feel that I am at a complete loss I must remember to honor this restructuring as creating something new upon the old. When my altar unexpectedly burned down, it was only the figure of a dancing Shiva that remained.

STRENGTH FOR THE SOUL: SENSUAL PLEASURES

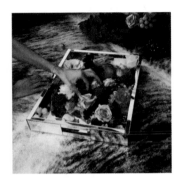

Every day for this entire week select a sensual activity. You may have your own favorite pleasures, or here are some other ideas of sensual activities:

- Take a trip to a sex shop and get yourself a toy.
- Explore the book *Slow Sex* or listen to a TED Talk by Nicole Daedone.
- Listen to sexy music, like Prince and Zero 7.
- Try a pole dancing class.
- Read good erotica such as a volume of *The Diary of Anaïs Nin*.
- Take a belly dancing class.
- On YouTube watch Annie Sprinkle on sacred sex.
- Share a secret with someone you trust.
- Go skinny-dipping, or be naked outdoors (without breaking the law!).

HEART FACT Sexual activity increases the pulse rate from 70 beats per minute to 150, making sex a cardiovascular activity!

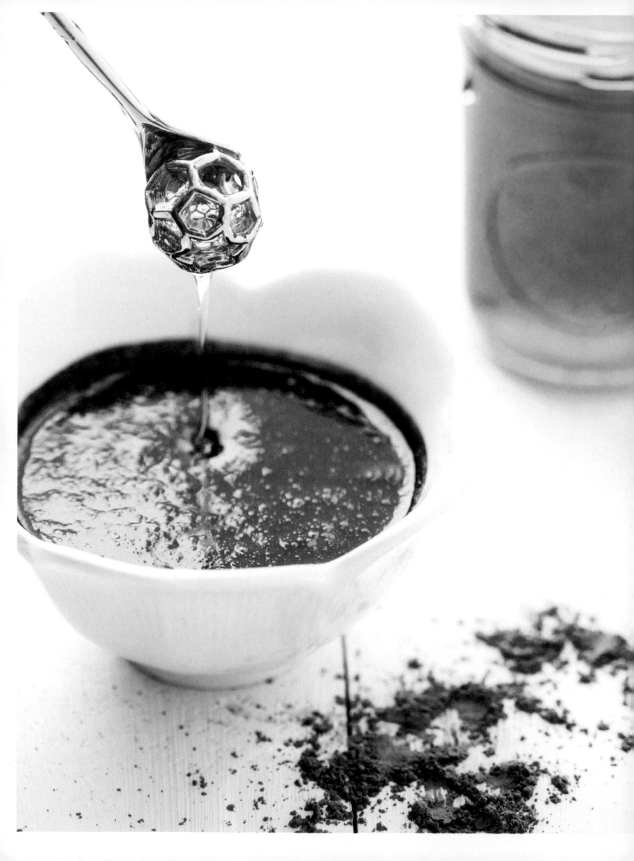

MMMMMANDY MUD

This incredibly decadent treat is made 100 percent from superfoods. When you begin to love and honor yourself, something amazing happens. You start to look forward to good wholesome healthy food! I guarantee: when you try this dessert, you won't feel like you're missing out on anything!

2 TABLESPOONS RAW
    COCONUT OIL*

¼–½ CUP RAW CACAO POWDER*
    (CAN BE CACAO VEGAN
    PROTEIN POWDER WITH MACA,
    CINNAMON, HEMP PROTEIN)

1–2 TEASPOONS RAW HONEY*

*Quantities to be determined by your desired taste and consistency. I usually start with these amounts.

In a bowl combine all ingredients in proportions to desired taste and consistency. (Note that the texture will change once it's refrigerated.) Stir until smooth and evenly folded. On a piece of parchment paper, scoop out 1-inch balls or drops and put in fridge. Let set until they harden—maybe 15 minutes. Eat as soon as you like, and store covered in the refrigerator for later, if you can restrain yourself from consuming the entire batch.

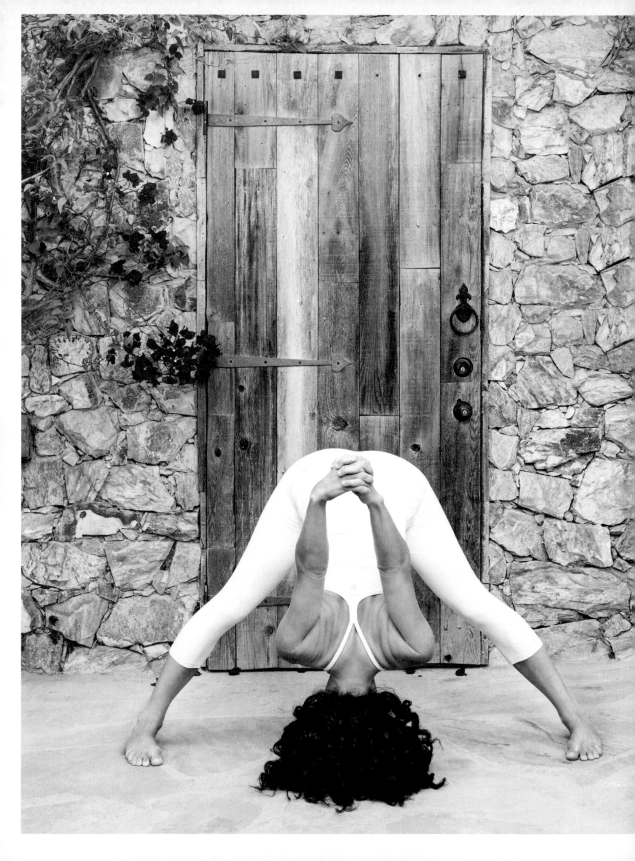

WEEK 9

Leap into the New Journey

You have come so far and have done such great healing work over these past eight weeks. You've worked to claim your solitude and reconnect with yourself, and given yourself the time and space to get to know who you are, what you like, what turns you on, and what you would like to shift. You've surrounded yourself with the nurturing that restores some sense of peace, and found the connection to your spirit. You've sought the friends or guides who supply you with the companionship and understanding that provides intimacy. You've given of yourself and reached out to help others from your wounded heart and found value and virtue in your pain.

"Love recognizes no barriers. It jumps hurdles, leaps fences, penetrates walls to arrive at its destination full of hope."

—MAYA ANGELOU

You have completed a transformational process, given yourself a fresh canvas, and are now prepared to leap into a new journey—because an entire world opens to you when a chapter of life closes. This is exciting!

You may say you're not ready. You may wonder how this new opportunity is going to appear. But I assure you, if you pay attention, you will hear a calling. There is no possible way that you could get this far on the path to healing without a spark and a flash of something brand-new. This journey takes you away from your ordinary life to experience the world outside your comfort zone.

One of the greatest things that you can gain as a result of losing what you have known is *freedom*! You can pack your bags without permission and set off on a journey of your choosing, initiated by you. It can be a call out to the universe, a "yes" to the future.

In a perfect world, I would say embark upon a literal journey, for that action may ignite a spark and give you a brand-new vantage point.

If you're able to take yourself out of your environment or plan a trip, there is nothing like uprooting yourself and plopping down in another location to shift your perspective and alter the course of your life.

I remember one of my students planned a cycling trip through Spain to give herself new perspective while going through a disappointing breakup of a six-year relationship. Boy, did it work. Not only did she release a relationship that was going nowhere, but upon her return she opened herself up to all sorts of new friendships and hobbies, and she became 100 percent more successful in her physical therapy practice. It seemed all she needed was a perspective shift. My little sister, just fifteen years old, had a similar transformation with a change of scenery. After our father passed away when she was twelve, she and my stepmom made a decision that she attend a boarding school in India. I was a little surprised by this decision. It seemed extreme to me. But, three years later, my sister emerged from her school at the foothills of the Himalayas with friends all over the world, a healthy first romantic relationship experience, and an interest in the environment, social justice, and the human condition. That was six years ago, and she's still really good at making new friends!

And then there's my dear friend Jennifer Aniston. She was incredibly resistant about going on location out of town to do the movie *Wanderlust*. But as life would have it, she ended up working with a great guy we'd met (on a trip to Kauai!) several years prior. Turned out that this guy became her dear friend and ultimately her husband.

It all goes to show that setting off on an adventure can be a pilgrimage toward deepening the connection to the true self and to others. You never know what might be right around the corner if you set out on an adventure and leave the rest up to the universe. There might just be the payoff you were looking for, or even one you never could have imagined.

After all of the soul searching and self-care, you can rely upon a greater force to plant a seed of courage in your heart to magnetize you to the next right thing.

✺ MY STORY

One of my most devastating personal losses came when I was just entering adulthood. At twenty-two, I had been a working actor for eight years. I had been on Broadway and in multiple television series as well as some films. All looked promising—my life was large.

Then, after a late night out at a coffee house, I cam home to find two men in the alcove behind the gates of my townhouse. Everything that followed seemed to happen in slow motion. These two men threatened to kill and rape me. Although the entire incident lasted less than thirty minutes, it would forever alter the trajectory of my life.

I tried everything from being agreeable, to wetting myself, to appealing to one of the men in a human-to-human way. Although that almost worked with one of my assaulters, fate had different plans for me, and I was forced to let them into my home. I was pushed upstairs by one of my attackers, while the other made a beeline for my room-mate Jamie's room.

Her muffled screams were almost inaudible, and I was told to calm her down. Once that happened, I was taken to my bedroom and forced onto my bed. My assaulter straddled my chest and arms and started choking me. As I began to pass out, my survival instincts kicked in, and I struggled violently, even as he punched my nose, eyes and all over my head. Each time he impacted me, I saw a flash of white. I was seeing stars.

Suddenly, from the core of my being, came a shriek at the top of my lungs. Before I knew it, both men scurried down the stairs and out my front door. Neighbors poured into my home downstairs as I met Jamie in the hallway. The moment I looked into Jamie's eyes, my heart sank. Although she looked intact on the outside, I knew she had been violated. I had been spared being raped, but she hadn't.

Several months after the violent incident, and two surgeries to repair my broken face, I took a five week trip to Europe with two of my dear male friends. I had been very gentle on myself and was ready to build my courage. It was just what the doctor ordered. I threw myself into the unknown, and embarked on a journey to explore other cultures and get out of my comfort zone.

Looking back, I would not trade the experience for anything. Jamie concurs. I learned so much about my character and my innate desire to live. I learned how to rely on others and ask for help for the first time in my life, and received so much goodness from people.

The trauma brought me back into my body and left me with a desire to be alive that I felt in my soul. After a period of thawing out from the event, my life became more vibrant and rich.

And so from the depths of unimaginable trauma and despair came a gift that stays with me today.

No matter what your tragedy, you can have a rebirth. Be open and say "yes" to whatever comes your way. You don't need to see the destination. All you need to do is take the next indicated action. Your heart has broken wide open, and so your world is a reflection of that. What treasures that may have been locked inside your heart are now exposed and shining, like the pearl from the oyster.

The key to moving into a new state is to keep on moving, so love your journey! The road ahead is paved with love, so just put one foot in front of the other.

SELF-LOVE CHECKLIST

YOGALOSOPHY FOR INNER STRENGTH program

- ❑ **Sunday:** Be Happy Yoga
- ❑ **Monday:** Back-to-Basics Yoga
- ❑ **Tuesday:** Cardio
- ❑ **Wednesday:** Bounce Back! Yoga
- ❑ **Thursday:** Day Off
- ❑ **Friday:** Let Go Yoga
- ❑ **Saturday:** Get Strong Yogalosophy
- ❑ **Heart-Opening Pose:** Wide-Legged Forward Bend With Hands Clasped
- ❑ **Love Movement:** Run!
- ❑ **Heart-Healing Meditation:** Japa Meditation
- ❑ **Love Notes:** Letter From Your Future Self
- ❑ **Ritual:** Create a Worry Box
- ❑ **Strength for the Soul:** Adventures and Experiences

MANTRA

Yes to life! My life is exciting and expansive. My journey is unfolding before me in a magical and surprising way.

TRACK OF THE WEEK

"Free Fallin'" by Tom Petty, "Everybody's Free" by Baz Luhrmann, "Elevate My Mind" by Stereo MC's, "Ain't Goin' to Goa" by Alabama 3, or "Where the Streets Have No Name" by U2.

HEART-OPENING POSE: WIDE-LEGGED FORWARD BEND WITH HANDS CLASPED

- Begin in a wide-legged stance with your feet about 4 feet apart and your toes turned slightly in.
- With a flat back, extend your arms out to the side. Inhale, lift your heart, and exhale, folding forward with a flat back.
- Reach your arms behind you and clasp your palms together, interlacing the fingers. Bring the arms up and over your head, maintaining the length between your head and shoulders. Breathe 5 deep breaths.
- To rise, press your palms together; on a deep inhale, rise with a flat back.

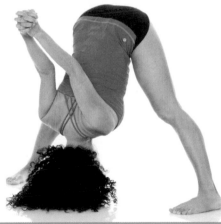

WIDE-LEGGED FORWARD BEND WITH HANDS CLASPED

LOVE MOVEMENT: RUN!

You can run on a treadmill or run outside. You can run on the beach or on a
track. It doesn't have to be a marathon,
or even that consistent. You can walk
for 5 minutes and then try running for 5
minutes. Running is amazing cardiovascular work. Have fun with it.

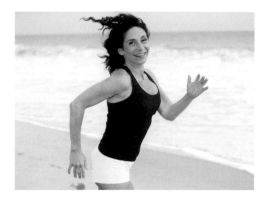

DENI'S STORY

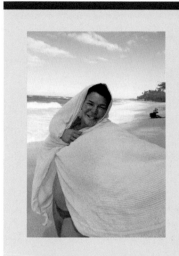

My twenty-two-year-old friend Deni Harrelson knows
all about setting out on adventures to find herself. After
growing up on the island of Maui and attending UC Santa
Barbara for a year, she found herself feeling a little lost,
as many do, going through the motions of higher education without a real sense of direction. Realizing that her
longing was for her sense of spiritual identity, which required that she go within to find it, she decided to attend
a Vipassana meditation retreat in Brisbane, Australia. That
path led her to Spain, where she walked the famous pilgrimage Camino de Santiago, followed by a two-month
trip to India, where she was confronted by many things she would never have explored
had she followed the status quo. She is currently on a ten-month journey to Sweden for
a Youth Initiative Program to help make a difference in the world. You'll find her beautiful
breakfast recipes on pages 293 and 295. Here is her relatable story on self-love.

• • •

Deni

I have been vegan my whole life and have been blessed to have such conscious, open-
minded parents who support me in anything and everything I do. I am now learning to

be more supportive and kind to myself, which is an ongoing process and one in which I am always being humbled.

From the time I was a child, I remember feeling a deep sense of compassion for others' suffering and always wanting to help people be happier by being as kind as possible. I lived for others and put their happiness before my own, forgetting about the importance of my own well-being. As I grew older, I felt the need to start focusing more on myself and my own happiness. I began to shut people out in order to protect myself from taking on others' problems as my own. I began to disconnect from the people I loved most and to numb my feelings by overeating. Ultimately, I hurt myself the most by doing this, more than anyone else could have. I broke my own heart by not letting myself feel at all.

Over the last couple of years, I have embarked on a journey of self-awareness and self-love by practicing Vipassana meditation and yoga, exercising regularly, and addressing my overeating habits. I am in the process of honoring this tendency and am currently doing a juice cleanse. I have already noticed a huge shift. I have more energy, I'm in a better mood, and I'm not so in my head all the time. By shifting my habits, I am allowing space for my heart to reopen and I feel much more nourished by love than I ever did by unconscious eating. In my experience, seeking vibrant and optimal health is essential. I am finding that I benefit both emotionally and physically by doing some type of liquid cleanse, to allow my body time to rest and regenerate so that my heart can bloom. It's amazing how attentiveness to what my heart actually needs is the key to being healthy and happy.

HEART-HEALING MEDITATION: JAPA MEDITATION

Japa is meditation using mala beads, which are traditionally used in Tibetan Buddhism for keeping count while reciting, chanting, or repeating a mantra. With each bead you roll between your fingers, you repeat a mantra. Mantras are often different names for God, with the understanding 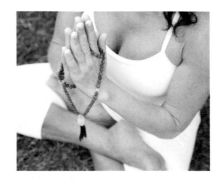 that certain words have mystical power. In Transcendental Meditation, they suggest a mantra for you. But a simple *"Om"* works, too.

LOVE NOTES: LETTER FROM YOUR FUTURE SELF

Write an encouraging letter from your future self back to your *now* self. In an earlier exercise, you explored sitting in the center of who you are today, and reassuring your child self that it all turns out okay in the end. Imagine there is a future you, and that future you knows the end of the story, exactly how it works out, what happens, and why things needed to go the way they did so that you could be blessed and gifted with all of the lessons and prepared for all of the treats that were up ahead. Let the letter reveal how amazing your life is in the future. Once you have written this letter to yourself, seal it and stash it somewhere. Open it in a year or more.

RITUAL: CREATE A WORRY BOX

Create a "Worry Box" where you can put all of your fears so you don't need to carry them with you on your journey. I made one out of a shoebox, but any box that size or smaller will do. It just needs to be large enough to hold little slips of paper. You can use it at any time or for any little thing that is nagging at you. You can be sure that the universe has you covered. This does me so much good when my mind goes astray and I am trying to think my way out of a problem, or when I am attached to the outcome. The universe is abundantly magical when we let go of the reigns and trust the ride.

Materials you will need:

- A box
- Collage materials (to decorate box): magazines, wrapping paper, stickers, old greeting cards, colored paper, etc.
- Feathers, glitter, beads, etc.
- Glue stick

Here's how to use your worry box: Whenever you have a worry, just write a note to your "higher self" or future self and begin with: "Dear Higher Self, please help me with ___. Thank you. Love, Me." Forget about *how* the problem will get solved, or what the outcome will be. Let the universe work its magic. You won't be disappointed. You don't need to go back and look, but if you like, you can unload the box in a year and see that, for most of what you were concerned about, all worked out.

STRENGTH FOR THE SOUL: ADVENTURES AND EXPERIENCES

Pledge to take action toward a bucket list activity this week. I've provided some suggestions. Feel free to add from your own list!

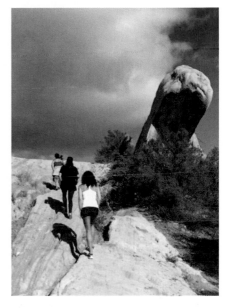

- Road trip, bike tour, yoga retreat in an exotic setting.

- Vipassana silent meditation retreat.

- Pilgrimage to India.

- Bicycle tour of a new city.

- Walkabout.

- Cruise.

- Astrology conference, or a conference on your special interest.

- Sign up for an art class.

- Sign up for a writing, cooking, or archery class.

- Take the guitar lessons you said you wanted to take.

- Find the hidden treasures of the city that you live in and make an adventure to-do list.

- Sign up to tell a story at The Moth, or another story-telling forum.

- Go river rafting or sailing.

- Sign up to do a marathon or a 5K.

- Get on that dating site you've been afraid to try.

- Mix it up!

HEART FACT According to *Harvard Health Magazine*, there's some scientific backing for the notion that regular vacations are good for your health. At least two large studies suggest that people who get away every so often live longer and are less likely to develop heart disease than those who don't.

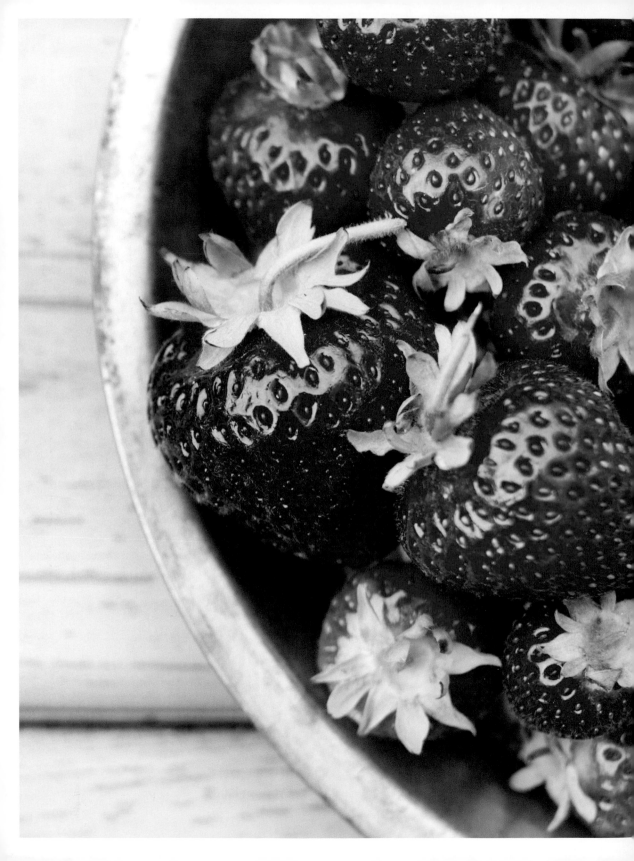

SOOTHME SMOOTHIE

Serves 1

This combination of fruits and flax oil often helps me to have a nice little release. You can add a little agave if you want it to be sweeter.

1 MEDIUM BANANA (OR 2 SMALL BANANAS)

1 TO 2 TABLESPOONS AVOCADO

3 TO 4 FRESH STRAWBERRIES

1 TABLESPOON ALMOND BUTTER

1½ TO 2 CUPS FRESH COCONUT OR ALMOND MILK

1 TO 2 TEASPOONS FLAX OIL

SQUEEZE OF LIME

1 TEASPOON HONEY OR AGAVE (OPTIONAL)

Put the banana, avocado, strawberries, and almond butter in a blender. Add the milk, flax oil, and lime. Add honey or agave to taste, if desired. Blend until smooth, starting on the lowest setting, gradually building to the highest setting, and then back down to low. Pour into a glass and drink with ease.

Recipe by Deni Harrelson

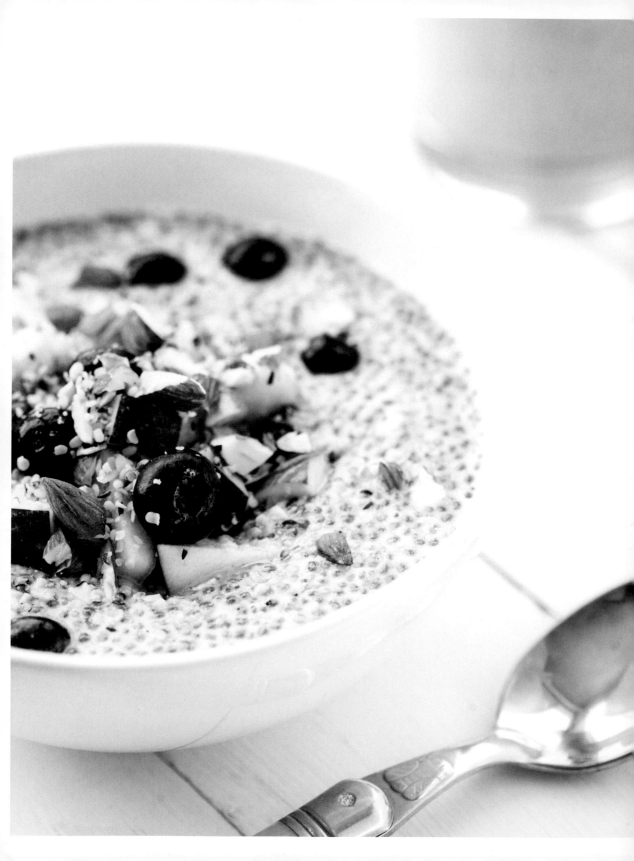

CHIA SEA

Serves 1

The flavor of this recipe is reminiscent of a bowl of cereal, but instead of all the processed grains, you get the benefits of whole foods.

2 TABLESPOONS CHIA SEEDS (3 TABLESPOONS FOR THICKER CONSISTENCY)

1–1½ CUPS ALMOND OR COCONUT MILK

1 TABLESPOON ALMOND BUTTER

1 TABLESPOON HONEY

10 FRESH BLUEBERRIES*

¼ APPLE, CHOPPED INTO SMALL CUBES

5–6 ALMONDS, CHOPPED

1 TEASPOON FLAX OIL

SQUEEZE OF LEMON OR LIME

DASH OF SALT

SPRINKLE OF HEMPSEEDS

SPRINKLE OF CINNAMON

*Feel free to add other fruit as well, such as strawberries, pears, cherries, or grapes.

Mix the chia seeds and milk together in a bowl, then add the almond butter and honey. Allow to sit for 5–10 minutes.

Add all the other ingredients to the bowl, gently mixing together with a spoon.

The most important thing is that you have fun making and eating it!

Recipe by Deni Harrelson

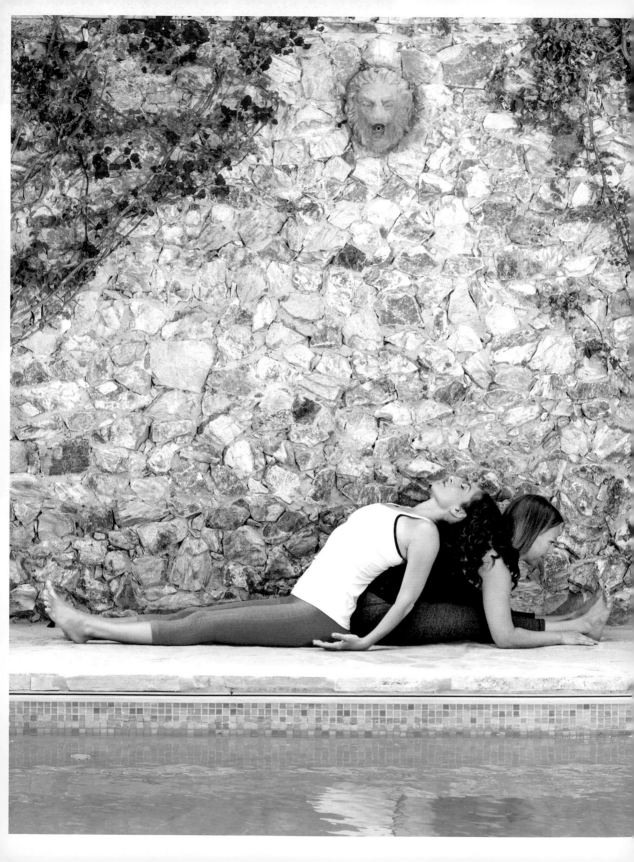

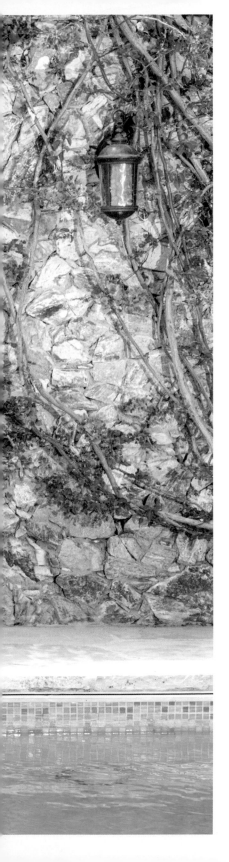

WEEK 10

Widen Your Circle

Did you know that friendship is literally good for your heart health? Studies show that people with a strong support group are 50 percent less likely to have a heart attack. That speaks volumes for the importance of finding the support you need just in terms of your health, but it's also a reminder that your true friends are valuable. The most healing and energizing experiences I've had have occurred within my groups of women friends. Group energy has an effect that transcends even as it empowers the individual. The perseverance you've had up this point can now be buoyed with the support of collective energy. This week, we'll go and find it.

> *"You are the average of the five people you spend the most time with. Choose wisely."*
>
> —JIM ROHN

Consider the law of momentum. Once something begins to move, the inertia of the movement will keep it going. Or consider the cumulative effect of doing an action repeatedly and consistently. As you enlarge your circle and gain the support of others, especially those who are also working on themselves, the energy behind that intention increases and the opportunity for a shift expands. When you connect with the collective energy of that widened circle, you're able to pull from a larger range of ideas, perspectives, and visions than when you're on your own. I like to think of each human being as a different lens looking at the human experience. When we each share what we feel, think, and see from our unique perspective, we can take a more well-rounded and thorough view of the subject. I'm sure you've heard of women's groups or men's groups where you can get together and share. When you gather with a collective group and participate, you contribute to a clearer version of the truth. That is the idea of "circling." Expanding your circle expands your heart. It allows you to be together in a way that's spiritual, supportive, and safe.

❁ MY STORY

In my family, when I had a point of view that was seemingly opposed to my parents', it was met with defensiveness. This left me feeling less confident to be myself. Luckily, my parents sent me to a school where each child was honored and given a voice. We were praised for our uniqueness and encouraged to explore the ideas and experiences that interested us.

It was in my school for experiential learning, MOBOC (Mobile Open Classrooms), that I first "circled." I was ten years old. MOBOC's "Feelings Session" was the antidote to the competitive and divisive setup in traditional schools. Each week, the group of ten students in my class would gather in a circle and, with the guidance and counsel of a grownup (teacher), we would be encouraged to speak about our feelings in the first person: with "I" messaging, such as "I feel this way," rather than blaming, such as "you did this to me." In doing this, we would clear up any emotional or relational issues that came up for us that week. I learned that I was respected in this setting.

This was my very first, but far from my last, experience with circling. As I grew up, I attended creative classes that embraced circling, particularly acting classes with very open-minded groups. It was in those rooms where we went around the circle so that each person could give a short share about what they were feeling, and ask for support when they needed it. Later, this morphed into several women's circles that I frequented. There was an especially powerful healing energy I experienced in the variety of women's circles I attended. Telling your story and being witnessed by the collective group serves as a magical salve. Being seen and heard has a power all its own.

Usually a circle begins with some version of a group meditation, asking for guidance, protection, and courage from a higher source that binds us in the highest good for all. Then we go around and each person shares, without comment or interruption. There is no right or wrong, and commenting on what another shares or giving advice is left *outside* the circle. This way a real feeling of trust can emerge, and individuals feel they can share whatever needs to be said without judgment. This can be timed or it can be free flow, depending upon what feels best for the group. In general, someone can be the facilitator, but part of the magic of a circle is that it *is* a circle. Nobody is in charge, and there is no hierarchy. It's not a ladder with rungs that are higher and lower. Everyone is equal and on the same level, each person is a part of it, and, depending on the number of attendees, you simply enlarge or shrink the circle.

I have attended circles as simple as a group gathered in a community center with fold-out chairs or as eclectic as a teepee with crystals and candles and decorated with symbolic objects. When I emerge from women's circles I always come away feeling stronger and more inspired by the variety of perspectives that I took in. Often there is a theme, like "trust" or "relationship," but it can simply be a gathering. In many circles I've joined, once the sharing is completed, there is some version of communing with others through a potluck or socializing. In one smaller group I was a part of, we made painting a part of the closure. In any case, the point is to find new ways to connect with your friends that feel safe and supportive.

Being part of a supportive community opens you from the closed place of heartbreak. It can be magical. There have been many times when I felt lost and alone, as if I were the only one who was experiencing emotional pain or isolation, and I heard another woman, a reflection of me, mirror back the exact thoughts and feelings that I was having—only they were regarding her and her experience. Often, when I hear the way another person is handling their experience, I hear a solution that never occurred to me before, or that I had been closed off to. Or sometimes I hear from a woman who seems to have it all, and when she opens her mouth, I see a different side of her. Someone that I thought was untouchable and had the perfect life—a long-term relationship, a successful career, who looked put together—was actually struggling with depression. It opens my mind, and my heart. I never know how what I share will help a friend in need.

Now that you are in the tenth week of our journey together, you may have established enough of a healthy sense of self to select your community. Plus, you've likely established a steady structure and routine that empowers you to be ready to be amongst larger groups of friends—and to integrate into the world. I encourage you to find a circle to join, or create your own. Love your lessons! Listen to your circle of trusted friends, and remember that hard lessons are just tough love.

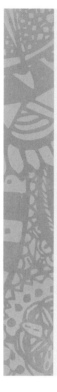

SELF-LOVE CHECKLIST

YOGALOSOPHY FOR INNER STRENGTH program

- ☐ **Sunday:** Be Happy Yoga
- ☐ **Monday:** Back-to-Basics Yoga
- ☐ **Tuesday:** Cardio
- ☐ **Wednesday:** Bounce Back! Yoga
- ☐ **Thursday:** Day Off
- ☐ **Friday:** Let Go Yoga
- ☐ **Saturday:** Get Strong Yogalosophy
- ☐ **Heart-Opening Pose:** Partner Yoga Backbend
- ☐ **Love Movement:** Dance Party After Your Circle
- ☐ **Heart-Healing Meditation:** In the Circle
- ☐ **Love Notes:** Write a Prayer for the Circle
- ☐ **Ritual:** The Circle
- ☐ **Strength for the Soul:** Items for the Circle

MANTRA

I am building a safe network of friends and supporters. Each person I encounter carries a different perspective of a shared reality. I am safe when I am cocreating and collaborating. I am supported and all is well in my world.

TRACK OF THE WEEK

"Dogs" by Damian Rice, or "If He Tries Anything" by Ani DiFranco, or "Sweet Nothing" by Calvin Harris featuring Florence Welch.

HEART-OPENING POSE: PARTNER YOGA BACKBEND

Let's take advantage of getting together in a group setting and do some partner yoga. It's fun and collaborative. You can do things you are unable to do when you are stretching alone. When you work with another person, trust and communication are important, so make sure to let your partner know if it's too much or when you need to come out of the pose.

- Sit back to back.

- Partner A comes into an extended leg forward bend, and reaches for their toes.

- Partner B leans on person A, using their body as support.

- Find what is comfortable and feels supportive. Feel your way through this at a slow pace.

- Person B can allow head to rest on A's shoulders as B pushes down and reaches for person A's feet. Or, allow the arms to open out to the sides, with palms facing upward.

- After a few breaths Person B lowers hips and Person A leans back as person B leans forward and lifts hips up into Bridge Pose.

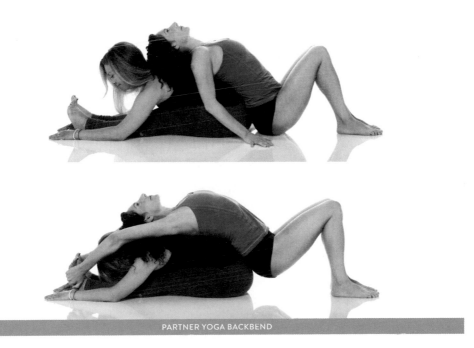

PARTNER YOGA BACKBEND

LOVE MOVEMENT: DANCE PARTY AFTER YOUR CIRCLE

There is no better way to commune and celebrate than to dance. My suggestion is to incorporate a dance party at your circle, particularly after you've shared. It will feel really good to move the energy through your body and be physical after you have been sitting for a while. (This may also be a good time to work on that partner backbend.)

ANDRÉA'S STORY

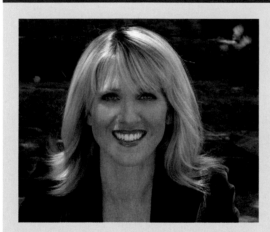

This week's expert is my dear friend and circling sister Andréa Bendewald, who created TheArtofCircling.com. Andréa has been leading women's self-empowerment and celebration circles since 2004. She uses The Art of Circling to create a deeper relationship to the authentic self, build community and support, and experience a sense of oneness that strengthens the human spirit. Her guidelines on how to give structure to creating your own circle are in the Ritual section on pages 305-308. Her story is reminiscent of my own friend/best-friend breakups, which are just as painful as losing a love.

• • •

Andrea

A few men, or shall I say *boys*, have broken my heart on more than one occasion. I can also state that I, too, have been the heart*breaker*! Mostly to psycho-obsessive types who lost their minds anyway, so those don't really count. The most subtle, and dare I say, the most painful heartbreak took place with a girlfriend.

She was one of my best friends; we knew one another's deepest secrets and had been through many lifetimes together. When the break happened the loss was real. She had stopped showing up in my life in the way "I thought she should." Pity party, table for one.

"What's wrong with rejection? What did it ever do to you?" Asked my wise fairy goddess mother over the phone. This felt like a trick question.

"She never calls me back, she only calls when she needs something, and she always assumes I will be available. She wasn't there for me when I got engaged! And then when I found out I was pregnant she had to leave town and "forgot" our dinner date. I mean, clearly, I was right, she was wrong! I was the better friend; she was the one not living up to her end of the friendship! I feel like crap and it hurt my feelings."

"When did it become her job to take care of your feelings?" Ouch. I wanted to whine and complain! Why wasn't my fairy goddess mother telling me how amazing I was and how mean and hurtful said girlfriend had become?

"Well if you don't like being treated like a doormat, then stand up on your own two feet." This hit me hard. Yes. Agreed. Why was I allowing myself to feel this way?

Our friendship continued to drift apart. I stopped calling her. I had planned a "breakup" dinner, where I would "let her off the hook" from this committed relationship, maybe we should just be honest and admit we were "seeing other people" . . . but she canceled, and we never officially broke up. We simply went our separate ways. I was devastated. I cried to my now-husband. He reassured me, "You'll be okay. You can't force a relationship. It takes two, babe."

He was right. I was better than okay. I actually began to grow up and to mature in the relationship department. Didn't matter that I was married! I began to focus more on my own life. I had been giving so much of my "best" to other people but not to me. I had placed a grand amount of importance, expectation, and unreasonable demands on this friendship, and she was clueless. It's a wonder the breakup didn't happen sooner. I began to breathe life into other areas of my relationships, with my husband, new women friends, and, most important, myself. I shared a lot about this particular sorrow in my monthly moon circles and had the support and understanding from a whole collective of women. My fairy goddess mother was proud of me. "You see, when your heart breaks, it doesn't really break at all, it simply breaks open."

HEART-HEALING MEDITATION: IN THE CIRCLE

When we are gathered in a circle for meditation, the group energy can be extremely supportive and energizing. As with exercise, we can often last longer and connect more deeply when we are surrounded by others who are doing the same. See the next page for some guidelines on how to circle!

LOVE NOTES: WRITE A PRAYER FOR THE CIRCLE

Write a prayer of an offering that you are making your circle. What is in your heart? What are you asking for and what are you releasing? Trust your inner guide to know exactly what to write and how to express it. Keep it simple.

ask the expert

RITUAL: THE CIRCLE

My dear friend and long-time circling expert, Andréa Bendewald, gives us a brief description of circling and how to do it. You can find her work at www.TheArtofCircling.com.

GUIDELINES FOR CIRCLING

These guidelines are designed to create a safe space for you and your circle to experience ultimate connection, radical support, and a spiritual awakening—and hopefully to enhance your healing. These are not really rules so much as guidelines that have served me well in my twenty-plus years of circling. Be creative and add your own as your circle grows and evolves!

Dedication

At the beginning of every circle someone lights a candle in the centerpiece and dedicates the circle to someone or something.

Talking Stick

We use a talking stick or piece. Whoever has the talking piece gets to share. One person shares at a time. We speak from the heart and we listen from the heart. There is no cross talk, advice, or conversation. This allows us to really hear ourselves speak, without the fear of being interrupted. Our egos get a chance to rest and our authentic voice/spirit gets to be heard!

"Ho!"

We say "Ho!" when we hear the truth being spoken. This is Lakota, short for "all my relations." Everything is connected. Saying "ho" doesn't interrupt someone's share; it simply lets them know they are connecting with others in the circle.

Don't Rehearse

When someone else is sharing, try not to rehearse what you're going to say when it's your turn. Be present. Truly listen.

Keep It Lean

Get to the point, the real essence of your share, especially if it's a big group.

Sacred Share

Whatever is shared in the circle stays in the circle. We can share our own experience from the circle. We want to refrain from sharing anyone else's story, even it is was a positive one. Please keep it sacred, even if you are sharing with someone who really knows the person—such as close friend or family. No gossiping. We get to practice nonjudgment and radical self-acceptance through the use of this guideline.

Silent Share

You don't have to share if you don't want to. You can participate by just listening.

Self-Care

There is usually a group break, so if you need to go to the bathroom, get some water, make an important phone call, etc., try to wait. But if you cannot, self-care is encouraged. But please, no cell phones in the circle.

Share First

Please share about yourself first before responding to what someone else shared. You can share how something made you feel or what it woke up inside of you, but we want to refrain from giving advice, or having the ego to try to teach in that moment.

Keep Circle Talk in the Circle

If you feel like continuing a supportive share you might say, "I'm really thinking about what you shared, it reminds me of a time . . ." But keep circle talk in high regard.

All circle talk should be done with love, compassion, and support. When a "Round of Support" or reflection is introduced, it is not a place for giving advice but a chance to support our circle mate. Lend support on the subject they shared. Support can be shared in the form of telling a personal story that relates to the person and situation they shared.

Emotions and Authentic Self

There is room for every emotion in a circle. Tears are welcome. Laughter is welcome. The shadow is welcome. The highest self is welcome. Wherever you are in your journey, sharing of your authentic self is what we are here to experience. Your truth may be the exact thing that sets someone free in the circle.

HOW TO CREATE YOUR OWN CIRCLE

Get a group of friends together—as few as four or as many as twenty. All you need is a space where you can sit in a circle and hopefully not be interrupted by the outside world. Allow for a good two hours; sometimes circles take flight and go on longer—you can determine the length as you go.

Think of your circle as a co-creation with the other members of your unique tribe. Choose a circle facilitator (a word that means "to make easy"), someone who will lead the circle from beginning to end. The facilitator is there to serve the needs and desires of the collective. Try not to be attached to the circle "going a certain way," but be open to the natural unfolding of what needs to take place for everyone.

- Choose a theme for your circle. What's going on in your life right now? Are you looking for partnership? Want to find a purposeful career? Are you looking to manifest more in your life? Are you craving deeper connections with yourself and friends? Wherever you are in your life is a great place to start! Every circle I have ever led stemmed from a strong desire within me to explore or bring something new into my life.
- Burn white sage to clear the space, and burn the same sage around each member of your circle. This ancient act is done to release any negative energy you might be carrying with you and allows you to go into the circle open and free.
- Once everyone has taken a seat in the circle, read the guidelines out loud.
- Begin by passing the talking stick and inviting everyone to share their names and what brought them to the circle. Then you can suggest a *prompt* or a question to get the circle going. For example:
- What are you most grateful for right now, today?

- High/Low: What's been the highlight of your past month? What has been the low point?
- Share a story about another woman who has been an inspiration or support in your life. Or share a story about how you supported another woman in your life.
- Share a story about your mother, a mother figure, or your own journey as a mother.
- After a few rounds of sharing you will notice a theme emerging from the prompt. Go with it! You can suggest more prompts to take the circle deeper or simply keep the talking stick going round and round until you feel the natural progression of the circle coming to a close.
- Next you can offer a witness or support round. Using the word "support" keeps us away from offering advice and keeps the circle more balanced.
- Another prompt could be: "What are you going to take with you from the circle? And what are you ready to leave behind?" Add a fun motion of throwing something imaginary in the center and then retrieving the thing you are taking with you. Adding action to words helps us remember what it is we are truly wanting for ourselves.
- Give thanks for the circle and everyone who participated. I love the saying "May the circle be open, but never broken"—the sentiment being that we take all the wonderful energy that was stirred up in the circle with us throughout our lives, until we can circle again and create some more.
- Enjoy a potluck dinner after the circle. It's a great way to continue whatever was stirred up! Which is usually a whole host of wonderful topics. Repeat the process the next month.

STRENGTH FOR THE SOUL: ITEMS FOR THE CIRCLE

- Crystals, candles
- Sage, incense
- Tarot cards, angel cards, Osho deck
- Cards of Your Destiny book
- Colorful fabrics
- Pillows to sit on (if sitting on the floor)
- Chairs or couches arranged in a circle (if not sitting on the floor)
- A light if you'll be reading something (perhaps information on the full or new moon, guidance from a spiritual text such as Louise Hay or the prayer of compassion from St. Francis of Assisi, etc.)
- Flowers, fruit, tokens—any offerings that make the circle feel bountiful and beautiful

 According to a professor of psychology at Humboldt University, people with social support have fewer cardiovascular problems and lower levels of cortisol.

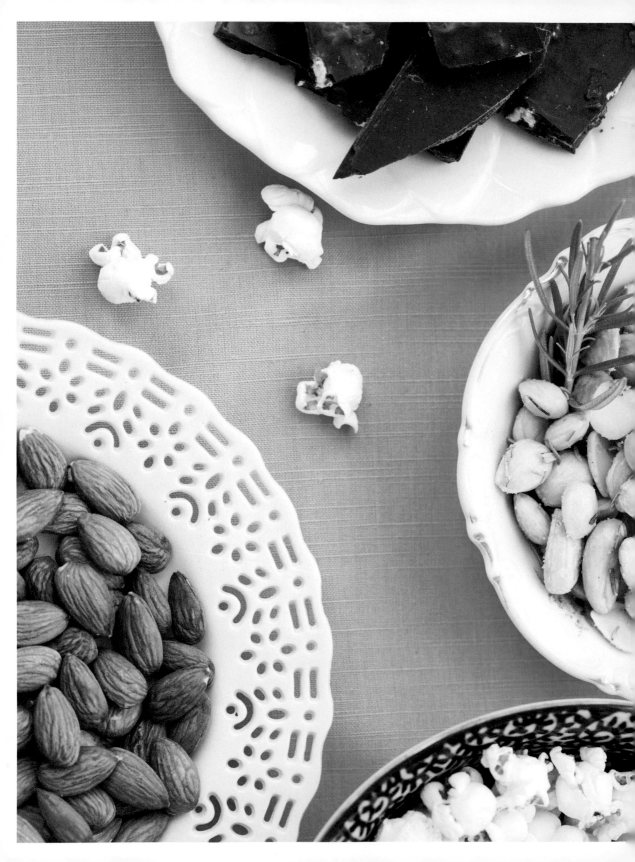

POTLUCK!

Create a treat to share with the circle for a potluck. Select from your list of heart-healthy foods found in the overview and prepare with love.

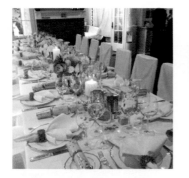

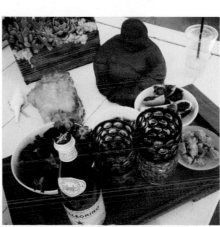

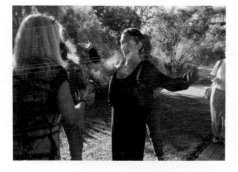

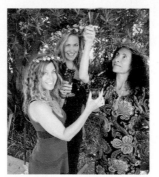

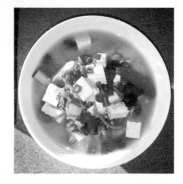

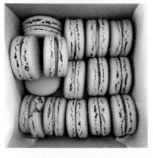

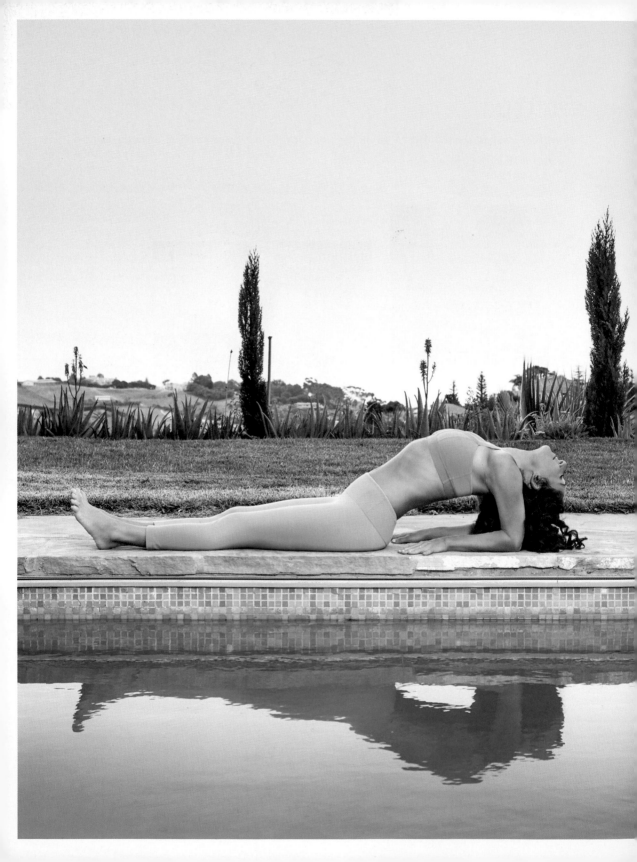

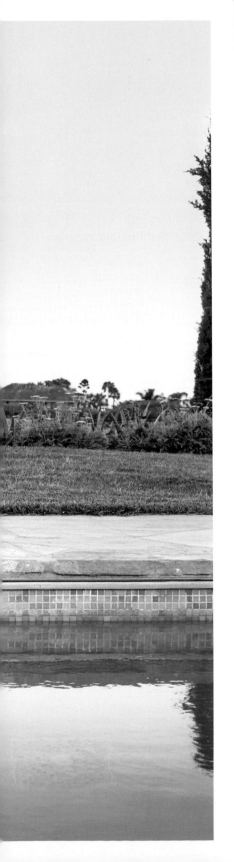

WEEK 11

Follow Your Heart's Desire

I n Buddhism they say that the second mind is in the heart. In this way, our sense of knowing is placed in our center of compassion. Likewise in ancient yogic texts, it is said that there is a cave in your heart, the size of a thumb. It is called the lotus of the heart, and it is where all true "knowing" resides. This is beyond the personal emotional heart, but the heart of spiritual truth. "Follow your heart" suddenly makes sense. The heart is the best placement of one's awareness. Trusting the knowing of the heart is a reliable source for connecting with what spirit wants for you. The beauty of spirit is that it is always present, reliable, and available to you. Spirit never leaves you. It is always with you, when you seek it. In times of great woe and strain, it can be easy to forget this natural and omnipresent force. That source is in the quietude of your very own heart. But all you need to do to connect with it is to become aware of it. And that's exactly what we'll work on this week.

One of the primary gifts you may encounter, as a result of the "unyoking" you've recently experienced, is the ability to get more quiet and connected to the inner workings of your heart. Inside that space, that second mind is the wisdom of your truth. Your true heart's desire is in alignment with the overarching force of nature. Within you is the knowledge of exactly what you're here to do and that your one job is to discover that. You are a puzzle piece and have a special place where you fit in that belongs to no other. You will not need to force your perfect fit—it will feel just right.

How do you heed that call? How do you get quiet enough to hear that voice? Certainly the movements you've been doing over these past weeks have led you to explore a self-loving state that allows you more space to be more of yourself. Seeking spiritual awareness is the key to having more spirit in all that you do. The mere act of seeking will reveal that spirit. What you focus on expands. It is really that simple.

I often think of how happy the universe must be when it sees me using my gifts. Using your gifts is a direct expression of appreciation. I imagine it's like when you give a friend a gift, say a beautiful necklace, and you see her wearing it. It brings you joy to see that she is using the gift you gave to her. The universe must work that way too. ___ly in the process of uncovering my own heart's desire. The first step is ___gh to recognize where I need to open up and give the love to myself. It ___ing my situation with conscious words and reigning in the wild mind ___ery of a meditator. I slow down, reconnect with my natural rhythm, ___hone my thoughts. I allow myself to feel and be responsible to feeling ___om that place, restricting myself from the old habits and replacing that ___ service to those in need—and then confiding in someone I trust, transcending my shame and expanding into an entirely new journey. I am rebuilding myself by connecting with my community, and soon I will heed the call of my heart. I'm unsure if I am able to put into words yet what my heart calls out to me. Small thoughts like: "Maybe you can fit an easel into your apartment," or "Maybe you can get a pet," arise. Or I just find myself in the right place at the right time. It's the voice that sends me back into hip-hop dance classes and has me suggesting road trips to Ojai or Big Sur with friends. Quite simply, my little urges and desires are there, and I am listening for clues. I ask each day to be guided to the people who are the right people for me to be around, and for the next right action to appear in my path. My intuition tells me things. I am listening. It's the same intuition that synchronistically thinks of a friend I haven't seen in months five minutes before that friend texts me. You know what I'm talking about, because these little miracles happen for you too.

So here it is: spirit is in a conversation with you all of the time. It's time to pay attention and join in to make it a dialogue. My personal daily ritual goes something like this: first, I sleep in a separate room from my cell phone. The frequency of electronics impedes the connection to spirit. It is imperative that you rid your sleeping space of all electronics if you want more connection to your higher self. I sleep with a rose quartz crystal in my hand. I use this crystal because there are very powerful healing properties in crystals and gems. Rose quartz is a very gentle stone that encourages self-love and self-esteem. Then, when I rise, I meditate for about 20 minutes. I then spend 20 minutes writing a "thank-you" note for the grace that I am given daily, plus ten good things I did the day before, and ten things I have absolutely no control of. I write a note, asking to be shown the way today, and I run any other unfinished business through my pen. If something is bothering me, if there

> *"Each moment in each day is a miracle waiting to be discovered, and when you are in flow, you will begin to see more and more of this around you all of the time."*

is anything on my end that I need to clean up, I focus on that. Once I see what part I have in the situation, it makes it easier to make a shift and then move on. I then read something spiritual, like a message that I can take with me in my day. You could call this my daily intention. I see it as a message from the universe to me. Next, I kneel on the ground and give myself to the universe, and ask to be led to the right place and to serve the love. I drink my hot water with lemon, run a bath, and am ready for my love movement for the day. When I begin my day this way, it reminds me to pay attention. I can remind myself of this at any time during the day. I start over at any point I need to. So, my primary concern during my day is to stay connected to my heart because that is how the universe speaks to me.

How many times have you had a call from your heart, or an intuition that you listened to? I want you to get more attuned to that way of living and being. You will find miraculous results. Each moment in each day is a miracle waiting to be discovered, and when you are in flow, you will begin to see more and more of this all around you all of the time.

MY STORY

Do you remember the fairy tale love that was going to rescue me? It took me almost three years to rid myself of the hurt I acquired from that first love. At the end of those three years, I started feeling whole again. Life seemed more exciting. Yes, I had taken all those hits, including the despair of my father's death that I described in *Yogalosophy: 28 Days to the Ultimate Mind-Body Makeover*. I took my hits well and I integrated them. Life was not without pain, but the resilience of the heart was its own reward for sure. I distinctly remember when I got over that original wound. I remember being led. I had my entire weekend open and free. I remember saying out loud to the universe: "Wow! I am so excited that the only thing I have going on all weekend is that I am teaching my class, and after that, I am completely open!" That was very unusual and felt so good. Only hours later, after my Spinning class, this adorable guy came up to me and started flirting with me (even though I didn't realize it at first). I have a rule that I don't open myself up to date my students. Oops. There he was and he was hanging around trying to get my attention. He even said, "Can you tell that I still want your attention?" I asked him what kind of attention he wanted and he walked right up to me and asked me to dinner that night. I knew I was free. So I took his number and we were set for dinner. Little did I know of the growth, love, and enrichment I would have with him. Cut to now, about nine years later. I am getting over that relationship. I don't know how long it will take me, and what will befall me. What I do know is that my heart is resilient and that one day, when I am feeling whole and I least expect it, there will be another person's open heart and my heart. I will be listening.

Love your community. Each day, you can attune yourself to the universal love that resides within the cave of your heart. This lotus heart is transpersonal and knows all. It is hidden within you. We are all connected to one another and move in love together.

SELF-LOVE CHECKLIST

YOGALOSOPHY FOR INNER STRENGTH program

- [ ] **Sunday:** Be Happy Yoga
- [ ] **Monday:** Back-to-Basics Yoga
- [ ] **Tuesday:** Cardio
- [ ] **Wednesday:** Bounce Back! Yoga
- [ ] **Thursday:** Day Off
- [ ] **Friday:** Let Go Yoga
- [ ] **Saturday:** Get Strong Yogalosophy
- [ ] **Heart-Opening Pose:** Fish
- [ ] **Love Movement:** Joyful Act
- [ ] **Heart-Healing Meditation:** Candle-Gazing Meditation
- [ ] **Love Notes:** Commit to Yourself
- [ ] **Ritual:** Commemorate Your Commitment
- [ ] **Strength for the Soul:** The Healing Power of Gems and Crystals

MANTRA

I am divinely led by my heart, and every day I make a connection with a power greater than myself.

TRACK OF THE WEEK

"Astral Weeks" by Van Morrison

HEART-OPENING POSE: FISH

- Lie on your back with your legs extended and your arms down by your sides with your palms turned down.

- Press down through your elbows, forearms, and hands as you lift your chest and arch your upper back.

- Tilt your head back with your chin up and your throat open so that the crown of your head is in contact with the floor. Lift your shoulder blades and upper torso off the floor.

- Firm your thighs and hold here for 5 breaths.

- To come out of the pose, press down through your forearms to lift your head slightly and lengthen the back of the neck. Slowly lower your torso back down to the floor. Hug your knees into your chest for a few breaths.

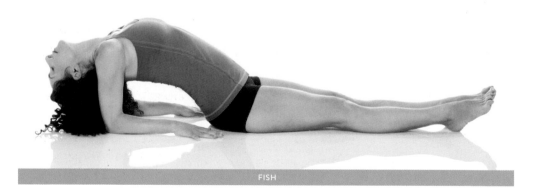

FISH

LOVE MOVEMENT: JOYFUL ACT

Take up an activity that you enjoy this week. Some suggestions: tennis, golf, rowing, paddle boarding, kite flying. Go back to something that you really love but have forgotten. Hip-hop, ballet, continuum, ballroom, square dancing, salsa. Feel the spirit move you.

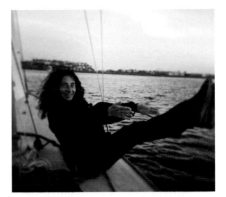

ELE'S STORY

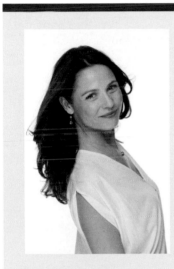

I have found crystal healing to be incredibly powerful through the years—a literal touchstone, particularly during times of grief and loss. This week's expert is jewelry designer and crystal connoisseur Ele Keats. She incorporates the magical, healing powers of crystals to create conscious jewelry for her jewelry store as well as in her own spiritual practice. You can find her crystal cleansing guidelines in the Heart Connection section on pages 322-324. In her story, Ele shares both how crystals have helped to heal her and ways to use them to move forward toward healing the heart, self-love, and the new!

• • •

Ele

As a child, I always appreciated the beauty of crystals, and the longer I have spent around them, the more I have come to understand their extraordinary and powerful energy. Many years ago, my mother gave me a crystal that was called a self-healer. This particular formation of a crystal is one that has been injured and that has healed over itself, meaning it was somewhat gnarled, nondescript milky gray stone, something you wouldn't notice. I remember thinking it was ugly and cast it aside for many years. Recently one of my best girlfriends, who also works with crystals, held it and said, "Oh my, can you feel how powerful this crystal is?" I closed my eyes and I felt into it and was moved to tears. This beautiful crystal that may not look so beautiful from the outside stores so much wisdom and an opportunity for self-healing. How many times do we cast aside uncomfortable or ugly feelings because they are so hard for us to look at? This self-healing crystal sits with me every time I am doing any kind of self-examination, healing, or meditation work, and it helps the process along in such a beautiful way. I am so grateful for my faithful friend that patiently waited for me to receive the self-healing. As the old saying goes, "When the student is ready, the teacher appears."

Some of my greatest teachers, and some of the hardest lessons that have transformed me the most, have come through heartache. Pink tourmaline is a very heart-soothing stone and has supported my own personal healing after a breakup, when I was experiencing deep sadness and loss inside my heart. Being that I work so closely with crystals and own a jewelry and crystal shop, it was very comforting to be in the space with these powerful guides. I picked up one of the larger pieces of pink tourmaline that we have in the shop and I held it like a baby close to my heart. The comfort and peace the stone provided was very supportive and nurturing during that time. Pink tourmaline helps disperse heavy heart energy, helps one trust in love, and is also supportive in embodying self-love.

Creating a love altar in your home is a beautiful way to invoke bringing in your partner and healing your heart. I created an altar in my space with crystals and a rose quartz lamp. If you are looking to call in an equal partnership, you definitely want to have crystals that are formulated moving the same direction and the same length. This will invoke equality and harmony in a relationship. Every morning when I wake up, I put my attention on the love corner of my home. It is, in my case, the rightmost corner of my bedroom, so I'm able to wake up and look over at my love corner every morning. Before I go to sleep at night, I hold my twin Lemurian crystal at my heart chakra and I envision my life with my partner. I hold the crystal as if it is my love and we are already connected. I've also written a list of all of the qualities that matter to me in my intimate relationship. I write all of that down and a few times a week I read it out loud as I hold my crystal and imagine us connecting. I then tuck this piece of paper behind the crystal on my love altar.

HEART-HEALING MEDITATION: CANDLE-GAZING MEDITATION

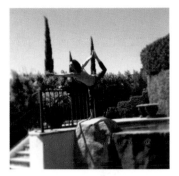

You don't need to own a crystal to focus your energy. Candle-gazing strengthens your focus as well. The mind is so powerful, but absorbing yourself in an object that mesmerizes you, like the candle flame, can help to train you to bring the mind to stillness. It will improve your ability to focus, and it will help to open the third eye.

Place a lit candle on a table three feet in front of you, at eye level. Sit in an upright, comfortable position, either seated in a chair with the soles of your feet on the floor, or on the floor in a cross-legged position. Take some deep breaths and begin to focus your gaze on the candle flame. Keep your eyes focused upon the flame, and try not to blink for as long as you can. As your thoughts arise, simply notice them, but bring your attention back to the candle flame.

Begin with 5 minutes; later you can increase the time up to 30 minutes. When you become more advanced, you may close your eyes and hold the image of the flame in your mind's eye. This is a wonderful practice for absorbing your mind. Take notice of what this does for your connection to your intuition.

LOVE NOTES: COMMIT TO YOURSELF

The journey you have begun has revealed much to you about what you need, and has shown you more of who you are. I've heard it said that what we are looking for we must become for ourselves. This week make a commitment to yourself. What are the things you have wanted? Write your vows to yourself. What promises can you make to yourself for the future? What are you willing to commit to? How much do you love yourself and what do you love about you? Say it!

RITUAL: COMMEMORATE YOUR COMMITMENT

Buy yourself a ring or another power object or gem, and during the ceremony use it to ritualize your commitment from you to you.

ask the expert

STRENGTH FOR THE SOUL:
THE HEALING POWERS OF GEMS AND CRYSTALS
BY ELE KEATS

HOW TO CLEANSE YOUR CRYSTALS

When you acquire a crystal, it is recommended that you cleanse and program the crystal.

STEP 1: CLEANSING PROCESS

Stones hold energy, and it is important for us to release it. Cleaning your jewelry and crystals energetically is very important, so you may use this technique for that as well.

To do this, fill a small bowl with approximately 1 tablespoon sea salt (preferably iodine-free) and freshwater. Put the crystal in the bowl of saltwater and place it in sunlight for 1–24 hours. Or hold the crystal in your fingertips under running water, clear your mind, and imagine light flowing from the top of your head, through your hand, and out your feet. Circulate the light from the heavens through your entire body and out your hand.

STEP 2: PROGRAMMING YOUR CRYSTALS

Placing your crystals in the full moonlight is a very powerful way to charge them. After your crystals have been properly cleaned and charged, take a shower in the following way.

Create a dry salt scrub. Place $\frac{1}{2}$ cup of sea salt in a small bowl with 1 teaspoon of water. Stand in the shower without the water running and rub the salt from head to toe all over your body. Say the following: "Water, please cleanse and release all energies, entities, and anything that has attached to me, and I release it into the light now and ask for complete and total healing, clarity, and protection right now. Please and thank you." Turn on the shower and rinse off the salt. You are now ready to program your crystals.

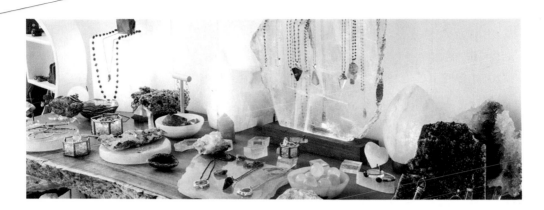

Once you are cleansed, take your crystal, place it in your hand, and speak your intention into the crystal. Trust that you will find the right words, and follow your heart. Just to offer some guidance, here is an example of what one might say: "Dear Crystal, Thank you for being of service to me and helping me manifest my desire. [Speak your desire], please and thank you, I empower you to support me and I ask for your guidance."

Crystals are definitely here to help us. I think of them as rock medicine just as one would take an herb or a plant. The rocks are able to provide healing, comfort, and transformation.

SOME CRYSTALS AND THEIR HEALING POWERS

TO TAKE ACTION: Amethyst, Fire Opal

SPEAK TO ANGELS: Celestite

NEW BEGINNINGS: Garnet

CHEERFULNESS: Amber, Fire Opal

CREATIVITY: Labradorite, Tourmaline, Garnet, Amber

COMPLETION: Aquamarine

HEART'S DESIRE: Amber, Hematite, Fire Opal, Malachite

HEART SOOTHER: Pink Tourmaline

HEART-HEALING MEDITATION: Sprouting Quartz Crystal

DEVOTION: Tourmaline

SOLVING DIFFICULTY: Garnet, Smoky Quartz, Tiger Eye

JOY: Aventurine, Fire Opal, Garnet, Labradorite

FERTILITY: Moon Stone

CLARITY: Aquamarine, Turquoise

FRIENDSHIP: Emerald, Lapis

ACHIEVE GOALS: Labradorite

INTUITION: Amethyst, Turquoise

LOVE: Emerald, Moon Stone, Tourmaline

SELF-LOVE: Rose Quartz

SPEAKING FROM THE HEART: Pink Kunzite

MOTIVATIONS: Amber

POSITIVITY: Malachite, Imperial Topaz

PROTECTION: Agate, Smoky Quartz, Serpentine

CONFIDENCE: Citrine, Fluorite, Garnet, Imperial Topaz

CLEAR THINKING: Agate, Citrine

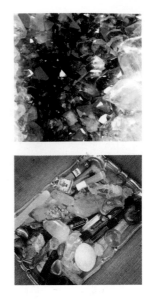

HEART FACT In a 1996 poll by the University of Maryland Medical Center, 50 percent of doctors reported that they believe prayer helps patients, and 67 percent reported praying for a patient. Although it's difficult to measure long-distance-prayer effects on a patient, current research suggests that there is benefit for those in ICU recently suffering a heart attack, as patients who were prayed for showed general improvements, had less complications, and resulted in fewer deaths.

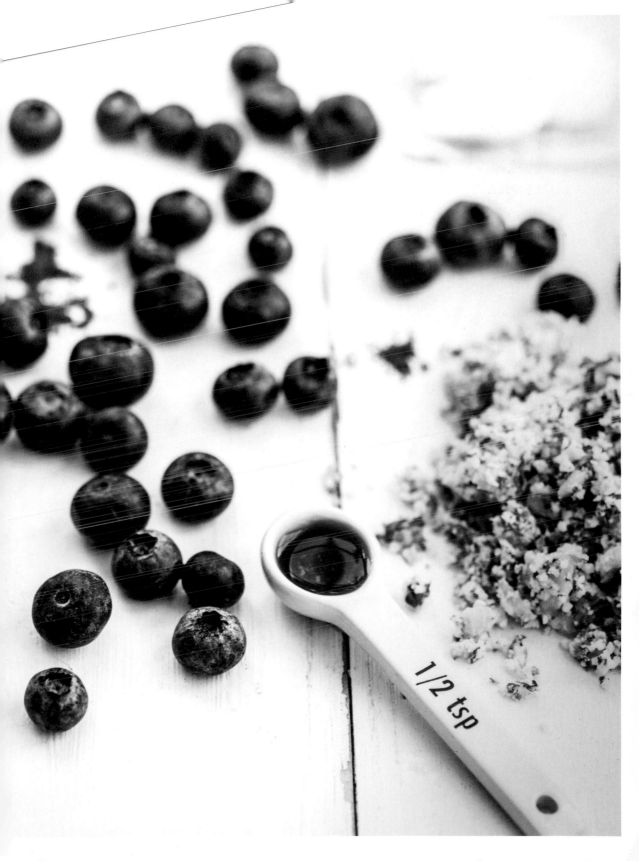

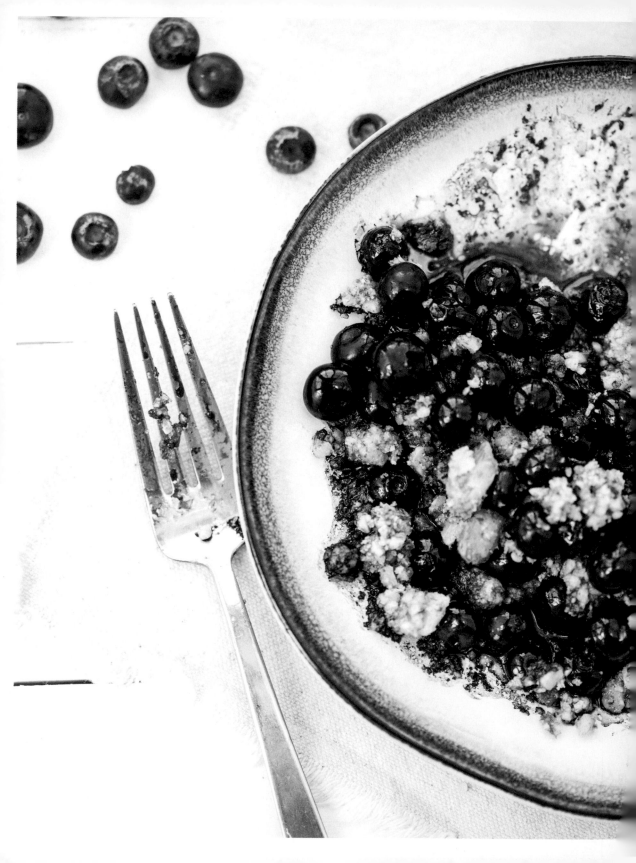

BLUEBERRY COBBLER

Serves 8

This gluten-free, dairy-free dessert is to be savored. Each bite is not only a tart and sweet symphony for your taste buds but is packed with the benefits of the miracle berry. Blueberries are associated with improving mental health, aiding digestion that can stimulate weight loss, and the combination of nutrients lowers cholesterol and supports your overall heart health.

4 CUPS BLUEBERRIES (FRESH OR FROZEN)

1 CUP ALMOND FLOUR

1/4 CUP COCONUT OIL

1 TEASPOON VANILLA

PINCH (OR MORE) OF CINNAMON TO TASTE

Preheat oven to 375°F. Coat a baking dish with coconut oil.

Place blueberries in the baking dish.

In a bowl, combine coconut oil, almond flour, and vanilla with your hands until crumbled. Sprinkle crumble over blueberries.

Cook for 20 to 40 minutes (20 for fresh blueberries, 40 for frozen).

Consume with pleasure!

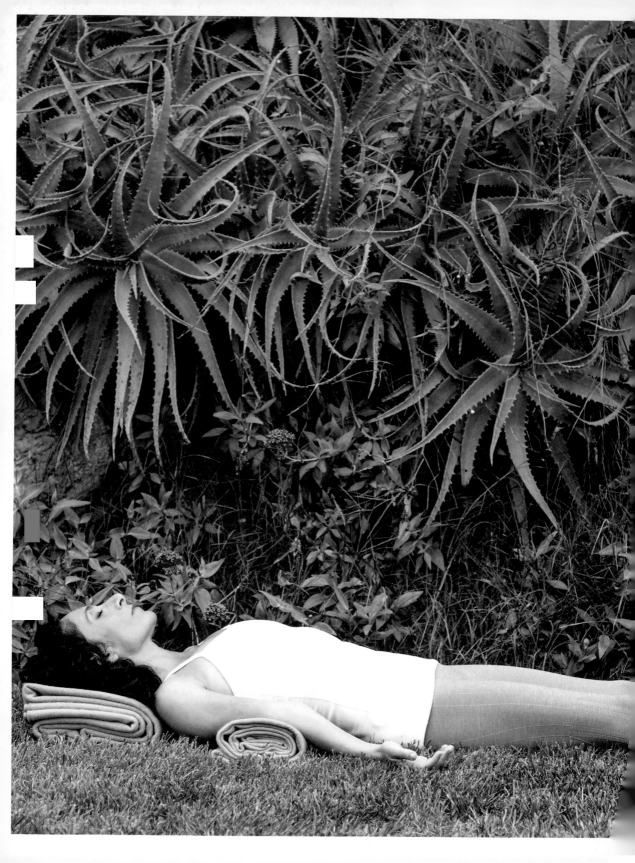

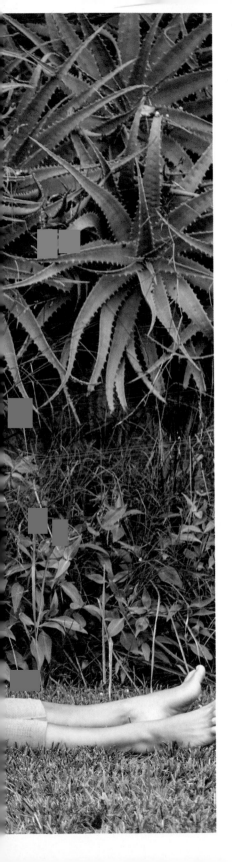

WEEK 12

Live in the Mystery

These past eleven weeks haven't been about "fixing" your heart; there's nothing to fix. They haven't been about solving a problem; there's nothing to solve. They've been about getting comfortable with and excited by the journey, which is ongoing. Your heart keeps growing and changing. Your heart keeps opening and becoming. Life will bring you challenges as well as joys, disappointments and achievements. It's all a part of the mix—the mystery that is life. Can you live in the mystery?

I remember being a child and wondering what I would look like when I grew up. I imagined that one day, I would arrive and be the adult version of myself living in the future. It would be all set and that would be that. I am not exactly sure at what age I imagined adulthood would be official. But I do vaguely remember, at about age twenty-five, realizing that the aging process was ongoing, and that I was going to continue like this, growing older, each year. So I am deducing that the age I was envisioning was about that, twenty-five. So here I am today, at age forty-seven. And it still keeps happening. I see that, inevitably, I am now a middle-aged woman, and one day in the not-so-distant future I will be an older woman. What I will be when I grow up is a continual evolution—as I become more and more of myself through life's twists and turns. As my face and body change, the "what will I look like?" question is evolving.

Like yours, my body is ever-changing and ever-evolving. The folds and lines of the trails of my life are etched into my face, the strands of gray hairs like the DNA that binds me to my elders, all twisted, spiraled, and thinning.

I have stopped awaiting my arrival. The children that I never had, the husband that never appeared, the house I never bought and decorated, the pets that I didn't adopt—my life has many unlived parts.

So I sit here, in this moment: a forty-seven-year-old woman, with all of my lines and wrinkles, in pretty good condition due to daily healthy habits, decent genes, and some luck. I share with you, from my modest one-bedroom apartment in Santa Monica, where I juice, do castor oil compresses, make tea, listen to music, and think about getting a pet or an easel. I share my experience, wondering if it is enough to share with you my secrets for overcoming heartbreak when I am not yet completely healed from my own? My life is imperfect. I still have a brother with mental illness, my physical health is in process, and stepfather is still struggling after his brain surgery. I don't have it all wrapped up with a nice neat little bow. I wonder if it is enough to say: "Life is a mystery and an ongoing discovery process, and you are in the right place, okay exactly as you are where you are"? I have to say "yes," it is enough.

Here is what I know: There is only one life that I am here to lead, my own. I chose this path in many ways, and in many ways this path chose me. Just today I sat thinking, *Would I have lived my life to this point any differently?* To that I say "no." I wouldn't trade my experience or the way I received my lessons here thus far for anything. So I sit, still halfhearted and unfinished.

> *"I wanted a perfect ending. Now I've learned, the hard way, that some poems don't rhyme, and some stories don't have a clear beginning, middle, and end. Life is about not knowing, having to change, taking the moment and making the best of it, without knowing what's going to happen next. Delicious ambiguity."*
>
> —GILDA RADNER

This is where I want to break the myth of returning to the whole heart. I have not been able to go through my life without my wrinkles, without the map of who I am etched into my face. Similarly, I will not leave this Earth with my heart untouched, as it was when I was born. I will leave this Earth with my heart a little bruised, some places enlarged, some parts with scars from being torn apart and from trying again and again. There will be some piece of me that still makes the same mistakes, and there will be places where I never learned and chose to believe, or where I was gullible because I preferred to have hope. My tender, broken, open heart still remains, and I willingly and lovingly lay all of that before you. This is my healing.

I was told that in this life, if I worked to heal myself, it would help others. My hope is that it is true. It's what keeps me going strong.

MY STORY

Today I'm reminded of a trip I took to India. I was on a silent meditation retreat, where many energies were surging and emotions were running wild and I was riding bareback upon my thoughts. At the end of the retreat, an older man who had sat in silence across from me in the circle approached me and said, "I can see that you have accepted and integrated your life experiences well." I knew that the reason he could tell this was simply by looking at me. My face tells the stories of the hits I have taken, but also of my magnificent resilience, which gives me a beautiful heart. I don't need to be healed, or perfect. What I do feel strongly is that I am unique, as I was intended to be. I have done my level best to accept who I am, the circumstances that life has offered me, and my ability to keep moving. Loving myself is a movement that I won't stop. I have found peace with myself in the face of the growing pains of the human experience.

I wish that my story had a resolution, like an *Eat, Pray, Love* finale. I can simplify it this way: eat well, pray for guidance, and love your path. I feel incredibly grateful to be able to wake up daily and move my body, to be open to others and content in my own solitude. If, through this book, you find your way to nothing other than that, then I believe you will find that is enough.

This week, love it all! Life is the yoga of coming together and letting go. This is a contraction and expansion, it is the inhale and exhale. I get to feel the beat of my heart, the pounding in my chest, and another chance to be in the mystery of love. And so do you.

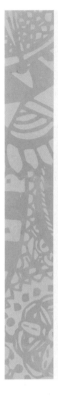

SELF-LOVE CHECKLIST

YOGALOSOPHY FOR INNER STRENGTH program

- ☐ **Sunday:** Be Happy Yoga
- ☐ **Monday:** Back-to-Basics Yoga
- ☐ **Tuesday:** Cardio
- ☐ **Wednesday:** Bounce Back! Yoga
- ☐ **Thursday:** Day Off
- ☐ **Friday:** Let Go Yoga
- ☐ **Saturday:** Get Strong Yogalosophy
- ☐ **Heart-Opening Pose:** Corpse Pose With Blankets
- ☐ **Love Movement:** Organic Movement
- ☐ **Heart-Healing Meditation:** Prayer
- ☐ **Love Notes:** Be a Poet
- ☐ **Ritual:** Draw Your Heart
- ☐ **Strength for the Soul:** Forward Bends to Relax the Nervous System

MANTRA

I am safe. Life is a joyful mystery.

TRACK OF THE WEEK

"Into the Mystic" by Van Morrison, or "Bold As Love" by Jimi Hendrix

HEART-OPENING POSE: CORPSE POSE WITH BLANKETS

We began the twelve weeks with Lotus Pose, the original yoga posture; now we complete it, as you would in your yoga practice, with Savasana, or Corpse Pose. This heart-opening variation uses blankets to support and open the chest.

- Use two blankets or beach towels, one rolled very tightly, and the other folded into a pillow.

- Lie down on the floor and place the rolled blanket horizontally beneath your shoulder blades. Rest your head on the folded blanket. Make sure that your heart is higher than your head.

- Close your eyes and remain here for 5 to 10 minutes. Allow your torso to release into the blanket.

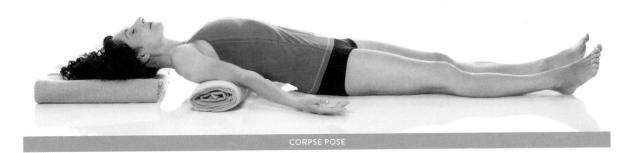

CORPSE POSE

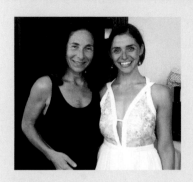

This week's recipes (pages 337 and 339) are from celebrity chef Vikki Krinsky, star of the series *Recipe Rehab*. Her contribution to the "Lean" diet option in my first book was invaluable, and her recipes are a real treat. Vikki's story sums it up in a few choice words, and I feel the same way each time I experience a cycle ending or letting go.

• • •

Vikki

My heart always breaks a little when I'm on the last bite of something completely delightful and delicious. Something as simple as almond butter swirled into Greek yogurt with chia seeds sprinkled in. Its smooth texture, rich taste, and surprisingly fun crunch creates a completely satisfying bowl of goodness. I suppose that same idea lends itself through life's precious moments, doesn't it? Those magical moments we may or may not tap into each and every day.

You carefully marry the ingredients together, knowing it will be the last time these flavors will give you their concentrated shot of colossal carnal joy. Your eyes close instinctively as you put the spoon in your mouth. Everything is in slow motion. You chew slower, feeling the food on your lips, your tongue, your teeth. It's deeply fulfilling and sad at the same time. Like a last sexual experience with a lover you know you won't see again, the last day of your brilliant vacation, or the last few seconds of your favorite song. Closing chapters, big flavors or small, can cause a lot of heartache. And, of course, we're not always given the opportunity to know that we're on our last bite of something so tasty.

As you smack your lips together and open your eyes, you smile, with immense appreciation for such an extraordinary experience!

Although I don't believe we can realistically treasure *every* second of the day the same way we do a bowl of creamy yogurt, I do believe we can slow down and fill ourselves up—mind, body, and tummy—with gratitude for each "bite" that we take in life!

LOVE MOVEMENT: ORGANIC MOVEMENT

What is your natural movement? Not dancing to burn calories or to get your heart rate up, but your organic rhythm. Whatever it is, revel in it this week.

HEART-HEALING MEDITATION: PRAYER

I have heard that, in the conversation with the universe, prayer is the talking to God and meditation is the listening. I have also heard that one of the best prayers you can possibly say is "Thank You." May this be your prayer.

LOVE NOTES: BE A POET

Write a poem about the mystery of your life. Life is nonlinear and poetry is a beautiful way to express that. Poetry is like painting with words. There is no right way to do it. So simply be a poet.

RITUAL: DRAW YOUR HEART

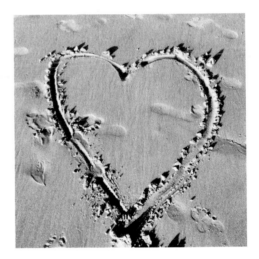

This ritual should be done in two parts. One now, and another in a month or so. Draw your heart. The first is a picture of your heart in the present moment. You may use any medium you like, but I use colored pencils or paint. Draw the best possible version of your heart today. Make it as beautiful as you can, don't hold anything back. Live with it on your wall for four weeks.

After four weeks, draw another rendering of your heart. This second picture of your heart is the way it will look in the near future.

When an old shamanic teacher of mine gave me this assignment, I didn't know that I would have to draw another picture of my heart. The first one that I drew was so beautiful I couldn't wait to share it. When I found out that I would have to create another picture, I was very disappointed: "But I love my heart the way it is!" While creating the second painting, I really disliked it, but I kept going. As I continued to work at it, all of a sudden I could see my future heart! It was beautiful. In fact, it looked a lot like my original heart, only blown wide open, like a flower transforming from bud to bloom. I've since learned that when I don't like my creation, it's because it isn't complete. Oh, and coincidentally, the two pictures of my heart preceded my first epic love affair. Do this ritual at your own risk. Expect love.

STRENGTH FOR THE SOUL: FORWARD BENDS

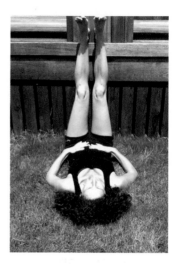

We have focused so much on heart openers in these past weeks. It's important to balance all of the expansion with poses to relax the nervous system. Forward bends allow the nervous system to calm down. You may select one of the forward bends on this list, or you may have your own that you like.

Seated-Forward Bend
Butterfly Pose
One Leg Extended
   Forward Bend

Wide-Legged Splits
Pigeon Pose
Legs Up the Wall
Reclining Butterfly Pose

HEART FACT Every day, your heart beats 100,000 times, sending 2,000 gallons of blood through your body, yet it is no larger than your fist. A good belly laugh can send 20 percent more blood flowing through your entire body. So the ability to laugh with life is the antidote to stress.

SALMON TARTARE WITH AVOCADO AND BAKED WONTON CHIPS

Serves 2—4

This flavorful blend is exotic, delicious, and full of nutritional benefits. Salmon is a great source of omega-3 fatty acids, which studies have shown may benefit heart health. This is also a great, flavorful way to try salmon in its raw form. Use the freshest, high-quality wild salmon you can find and eat to your heart's content. The avocado adds a creamy texture and the wontons will give it a crunch!

³/₄ POUND GRADE-A SALMON, ABOUT 1¹/₂ INCHES THICK

1 TABLESPOON OR 10 SPRAYS OF LIQUID AMINOS

1 TEASPOON SESAME OIL

1 AVOCADO, DICED

¹/₂ JALAPENO, SEEDED AND FINELY DICED

1 TEASPOON FLAXSEED OIL

¹/₄ TEASPOON FRESHLY GRATED GINGER

5 WONTON WRAPPERS

COCONUT OIL SPRAY

¹/₄ TEASPOON GROUND CUMIN

¹/₄ TEASPOON CHIA SEEDS

1 TABLESPOON SESAME SEEDS, WHITE OR BLACK

SPECIAL EQUIPMENT

ONE 2- TO 3-INCH RING MOLD

Preheat the oven to 350°F.

Start by cutting salmon in half, lengthwise. Dice the two halves into bite-size pieces.

In a bowl, place the salmon, liquid aminos, and sesame oil. Let the salmon marinate while you prepare the rest of the ingredients.

In a separate bowl, place the avocado, jalapeno, flaxseed oil, and ginger. Gently mix everything together; be careful not to break up the avocado too much.

Cut five wonton wrappers in half diagonally to produce ten wonton triangles. Place the wonton triangles on a baking sheet. Spray each side of the triangles with coconut oil spray, then sprinkle each side with a dash of ground cumin followed by a dash of chia seeds.

Cook the wonton triangles in the oven for 6–8 minutes total, 3–4 minutes on each side, until they are brown and crispy on both sides. Watch them carefully as they bake; they can burn easily.

To assemble the salmon tartare: place the ring mold on a serving dish. Spoon one-tenth of the avocado mixture in the bottom of the mold. Top with one-tenth of the salmon. Sprinkle with sesame seeds. Repeat the process with the remainder of the avocado, salmon, and sesame seeds. Carefully lift the ring mold to reveal a perfect mound of avocado and salmon. Serve with the baked wonton triangles.

Enjoy scooping up each delicious bite.

Recipe by Vikki Krinsky

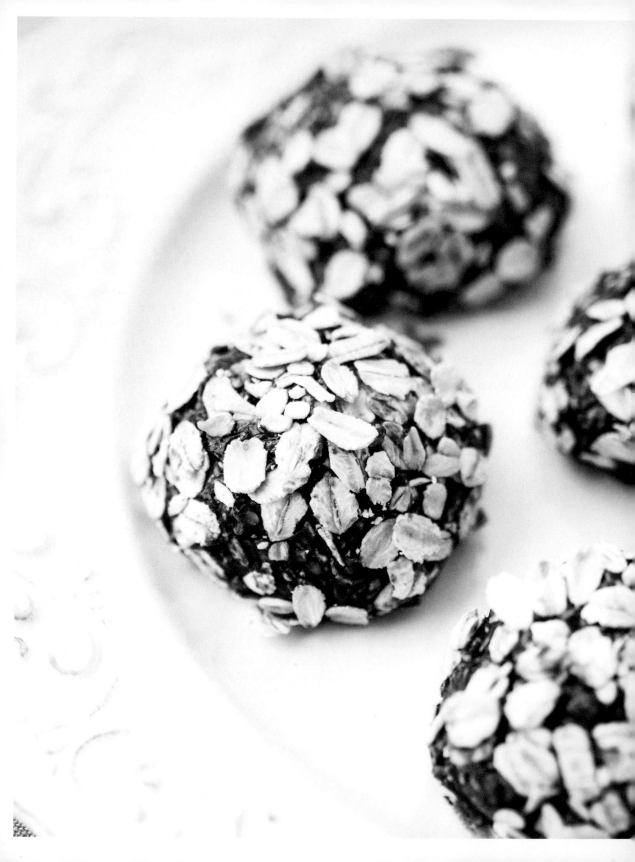

CHOCOLATE ALMOND OAT BALLS

Serves 4—6

Tying into the "joyful mystery" of this week's theme, share these yummy treats with a friend, and watch as they light up and wonder what's in your secret recipe! Delight in keeping it a secret that your seemingly sinful treat is 100 percent heart-healthy.

1 CUP ROLLED OATS

¼ CUP UNSWEETENED COCOA POWDER

2 TABLESPOONS CHIA SEEDS

2 TABLESPOONS FLAX SEEDS

2 TABLESPOONS HEMP SEEDS

1 CUP UNSALTED ALMOND BUTTER

¼ CUP HONEY (OR TO TASTE)

1 TABLESPOON VANILLA EXTRACT

¼ TO ½ CUP WATER (DEPENDING ON DESIRED THICKNESS)

In a medium-size bowl, add the rolled oats, cocoa powder, chia, flax, and hemp.

In a small saucepan over medium heat, add the almond butter, honey, and vanilla extract until fully combined and just heated through. Add water to your desired consistency and stir quickly until smooth. Pour over the dry ingredients and mix well.

Place the mixture in the fridge to cool, 10–15 minutes. Once cooled, roll the mixture into bite-size balls and store in an airtight container in the fridge for up to 5 days.

Recipe by Vikki Krinsky

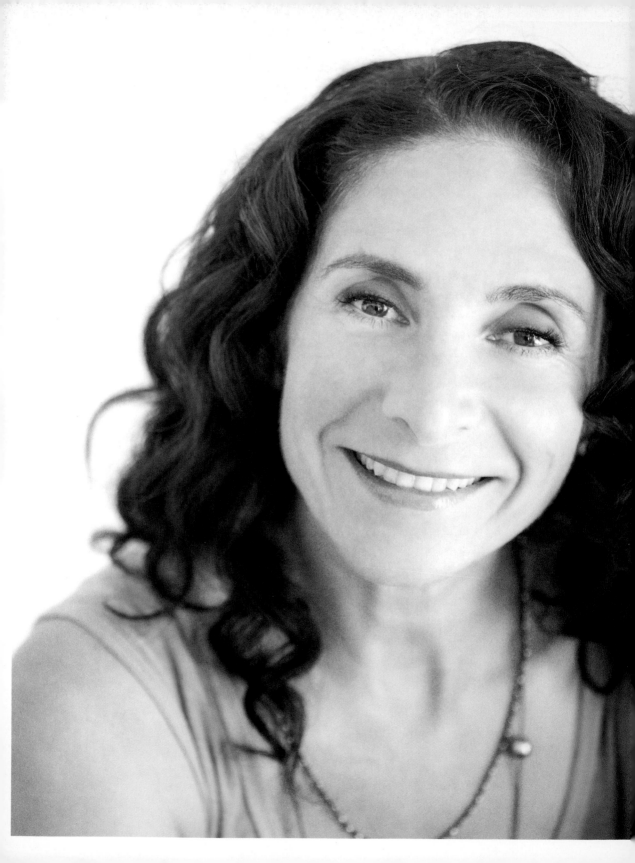

ACKNOWLEDGMENTS

It takes a village to create a book. I am so grateful for my amazing tribe who supported me through writing this book. My editors: Jenni Anspach, Lauren Childs, Erika Lenkert, Krista Lyons, and Laura Mazer. My visionaries: my trusted photographer Javiera Estrada and her team, Eric Charles, Michael Kinsey, and Sera Lindsey. Makeup artist Glen Alen and wardrobe gal Jill McDonald. Book designers Tabitha Lahr and Jane Musser. My powerhouse agent Jane Dystel for keeping me productive. My contributing experts: Laura Amazzone, Andréa Bendewald, Melissa Costello, Lauren Haas, Deni Montana Harrelson, Linda Ingber, Ele Keats, Vikki Krinsky, Persephenie Lea, Sarah Romotsky, and Alexis Smart. My familial relations: Dave, Naoko, Kailee, Stephen, Max, Megan, and the rest! My supportive sisters, new and old: Amy, Cynthia, Dawn, Elle, Gabrielle, Helen, Jamie, Jen, Jenny, Joely, Julie, Kate, Kay, Kristin, Laura, Lili, Liza, Mary, Mimi, Nadine, Natasha, Ricki, Sandra, Talia, Tonya, and Tricia Leigh; and my brothers from another mother: Bryan, Jon, Rich, Steve, Tom—and to those I am surely forgetting. A big thanks to the healers who helped me this year: Brian Campbell, Dawn DeSylvia, Ellen Heed, Gleah Powers, Gary Strauss, Tamara Trebilcock, and more. To all those who have broken my heart: I love you still; you are always in my heart and thank you! To the two strongest women I know: my mom, Chava Luba, and my grandma, Bubbie Sonia, who will skim this book looking for her name. Yes to that! Yes to life! Yes to love!

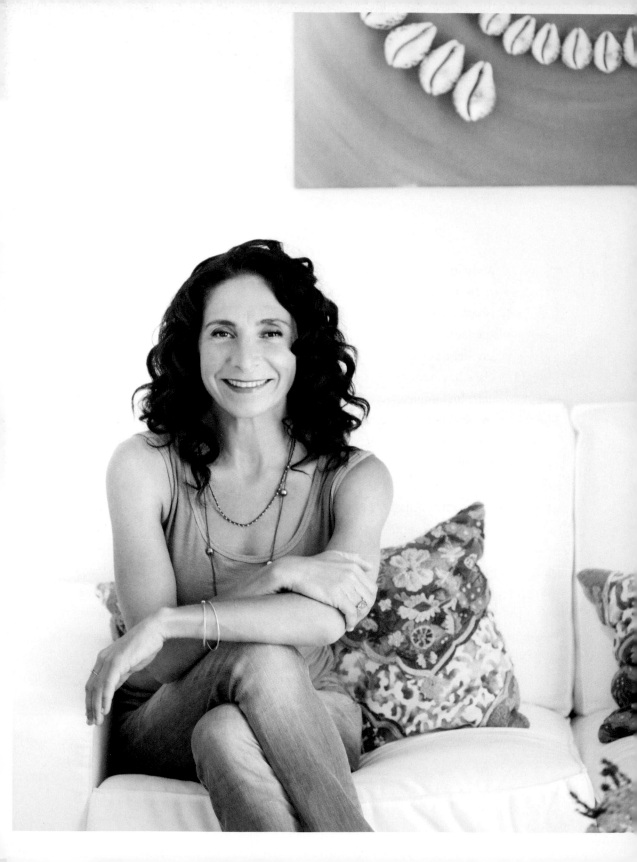

ABOUT THE AUTHOR

Mandy Ingber, the *New York Times* best-selling author of *Yogalosophy: 28 Days to the Ultimate Mind-Body Makeover* and creator of the yoga-hybrid DVD *Yogalosophy*, is a celebrity fitness and wellness expert. Her twenty years of teaching experience have attracted such clients as Jennifer Aniston, Kate Beckinsale, Helen Hunt, Jennifer Meyer, and Brooke Shields.

Mandy's class has been awarded "Best of LA" in *Daily Candy, LA Weekly,* and *Los Angeles Magazine*. Ingber is an event headliner for such events as the Boston Red Sox Foundation's FenwaYoga, People Magazine's A-List Workout, and more. She has been a spokesperson for companies such as Silk Soymilk and a contributing fitness and wellness advisor on multiple platforms, including *Health,* POPSUGAR, *SELF* magazine, *Shape, USA Today, Women's Health,* and Yahoo! Mandy is a fitness blogger for *E! Online* and www.People.com and is featured regularly in: *Elle, Glamour, Harper's Bazaar, InStyle, Los Angeles Magazine, O, The Oprah Magazine, People, SELF, Us Weekly, Vanity Fair, Vogue,* and more. Television appearances include *Access Hollywood, E! News, Fox Extra, Good Day L.A., Good Morning America,* the *Chelsea Lately* show, and the *TODAY* show, among others. Mandy is also on the advisory committee for the Cancer Prevention Clinic at the Margie Petersen Breast Center at Providence Saint John's Health Center. Prior to her career in fitness, Ingber performed on Broadway in the original company of *Brighton Beach Memoirs*, played Annie Tortelli on the all-time-favorite series *Cheers*, and is forever remembered for her famous rap in the cult classic *Teen Witch*.

Mandy Ingber teaches annually at the Omega Institute for Holistic Studies and at independent yoga studios. Follow her on Twitter, Facebook, Instagram, and You Tube. You can find her first book and DVD on Amazon and in stores. For more of Mandy visit www.MandyIngber.com.

INDEX

Happy Cow Pose, 49

Harrelson, Deni, 288–289, 293, 295

Harvard Health Magazine, 291

heart beauty treatments, 264

heart chakra *(anahata),* 17, 166, 167

Heart Forgiveness with a Parent
    meditation, 214–215

heart masks, 264

Heart-Melting Pose, 243–244

heart-opening poses, 159–160, 176–
    177, 194, 211–212, 229–230, 243–
    244, 260, 273, 287, 301, 318, 333

Heart Pulse with Mudra meditation, 232

heart space, 223–237

Heart Thumping, 246

Hepburn, Audrey, 269

hikes, 177–178

hugs, 215

Hurst, Helen, 225–226

hydration, 21–22

hygiene, 250–251

I

In the Circle meditation, 304

Ingber, Linda, 195–196

interval training (Wednesday), 31,
    88–113

intimacy, 269–281

Iysengar, B. K. S., 6

J

Japa meditation, 289

journey, 283–295

joyful acts, 319

Jumping Jacks, 94

Jumping Lunges, 44

K

Keats, Ele, 319–320, 322–324

kirtans, 233–234

Knee-In to Three-Legged Dog, 75

Knee Kick-Up, 101

Kneeling-Forward Arm Raises, 140

Krinsky, Vikki, 334, 337, 339

Krishna Das, 233

L

laughing, 216–217

Lea, Persephenie, 261, 264

Left-Side Jacks, 95

Leg-Back Jack, 105

Leg Straight-Up Sit-Ups, 108

Legs-Split Sit-Ups, 108

Lenkert, Erika, 162–163, 169

Light on Yoga, 6

Locust Pose, 73

Lotus Pose, 159–160

love movements, 9, 161–162, 177–178,
    195, 213, 231, 244, 261, 274, 288,
    302, 319, 335

love notes, 9, 165, 181–182, 198, 215,
    233, 246, 262, 278, 290, 304, 321,
    335

Low Lunge, 57

SELECTED TITLES FROM SEAL PRESS

Yogalosophy: 28 Days to the Ultimate Mind-Body Makeover, by Mandy Ingber. $20, 978-1-58005-445-4. In *Yogalosophy®,* Ingber—one of the most sought-after fitness and wellness advisors in Los Angeles—offers up a unique 28-day plan to help readers achieve healthier bodies and happier minds.

Super You: Release Your Inner Superhero, by Emily V. Gordon. $16.00, 978-1-58005-575-8. *Super You* is a fun, friendly, and unabashedly geeky guide to becoming the superhero of your own extraordinary life. With activities in every chapter to help identify each person's superpowers and personal kryptonite—and weapons against it—*Super You* is the perfect sidekick for every growing hero, empowering everyday people to transform into the most kick-ass versions of themselves.

Break Free from the Divortex: Power Through Your Divorce and Launch Your New Life, by Christina Pesoli. $17.00, 978-1-58005-535-2. Packed with no-nonsense advice and practical survival tips, *Break Free from the Divortex* offers advice from someone who can do more than settle your case. Christina Pesoli is a professional divorce coach and an attorney who acts as therapist, lawyer, and best friend, all rolled into one relatable guide.

Nalini Method: 7 Workouts for 7 Moods, by Rupa Mehta. $22.00, 978-1-58005-599-4. Rupa brings her revolutionary techniques for shedding emotional weight and achieving balance of body and mind to the wider world with a gorgeous and fun full-color book. *The Nalini Method* is an innovative mood-based fitness plan that fuses yoga, Pilates, strengthening exercises, and barre work to help participants transform both mind and body.

How to Break Up With Anyone: Letting Go of Friends, Family, and Everyone In-Between, by Jamye Waxman, $16, 978-1-58005-597-0. Relationship expert Jamye Waxman has written a much-needed guide to every step of a non-romantic breakup. *How to Break Up With Anyone* provides the tools for anyone to initiate a breakup, the encouragement to get through it, and the wisdom to recognize that they don't have to settle for anything less than productive, healthy relationships.

We Hope You Like This Song: An Over Honest Story about Friendship, Death, and Mix Tapes, by Bree Housley. $16.00, 978-1-58005-431-7. Sweet, poignant, and yet somehow laugh-out-loud funny, *We Hope You Like This Song* is a touching story of love, loss, and the honoring of a friendship after it's gone.

Find Seal Press Online

www.SealPress.com | www.Facebook.com/SealPress | Twitter: @SealPress